PLEASURE HEALING

MINDFUL PRACTICES & SACRED SPA RITUALS FOR SELF-NURTURING

MARY BETH JANSSEN

NEW HARBINGER PUBLICATIONS, INC.

Publisher's Note

This publication is designed to provide accurate and authoritative information in regard to the subject matter covered. It is sold with the understanding that the publisher is not engaged in rendering psychological, financial, legal, or other professional services. If expert assistance or counseling is needed, the services of a competent professional should be sought.

Distributed in Canada by Raincoast Books

Copyright © 2009 by Mary Beth Janssen
New Harbinger Publications, Inc.
5674 Shattuck Avenue
Oakland, CA 94609
www.newharbinger.com

Cover design by Amy Shoup; Text design by Amy Shoup and Michele Waters-Kermes; Acquired by Jess O'Brien;
Edited by Nelda Street

Printed in the United States of America

Library of Congress Cataloging-in-Publication Data

Janssen, Mary Beth.
  Pleasure healing : mindful practices and sacred spa rituals for self-nurturing / Mary Beth Janssen.
      p. cm.
  Includes bibliographical references.
  ISBN-13: 978-1-57224-574-7 (pbk. : alk. paper)
  ISBN-10: 1-57224-574-3 (pbk. : alk. paper) 1. Relaxation. 2. Meditation. 3. Yoga. 4. Pleasure--Health aspects. I. Title.
  RA785.J36 2009
  613.7'92--dc22

                              2008039810

1   10   09

     9   8   7   6   5   4   3   2   1   First printing

To my beloved James. Thanks for your unending support. To my wonderful family, especially my dear parents, Hubert and Nelly. You are such a blessing.

CONTENTS

Acknowledgements

I'd like to thank all my friends at New Harbinger for their belief in and support of my message. To Wendy Millstein for our serendipitous connection. To Jess O'Brien and the many others who helped to bring this book to fruition, giving it a beautiful look and feel. And my utmost gratitude to Jess Beebe and Nelda Street for your inspired editorial guidance.

My deep appreciation to dear friends and mentors alike for your inspiration, support and guidance especially Horst M. Rechelbacher, Deepak Chopra, M.D., David Simon, M.D., Max Simon, Gay Hendricks, Ph.D, Deborah Szekely, Candace Pert, Ph.D, Herbert Benson, M.D., Samuel Epstein, M.D., Mary Bemis, Beverly Maloney-Fischback, Julia Fenster, Rod Stryker, Ram Dass, Arielle Ford, Joseph Mercola, D.O., Francis Moore Lappe and Anna Lappe (`over the e), Gabrielle Roth, Ronnie Cummins, Kenny Ausubel and Nina Simons, Ted Ning, Marnie Morrione, Bianca Alexander.

And to the wise women, or shall I say goddesses, in my life Bea Sochor, Vi Nelson, Leslie Pace, Susan Macleary, Mary

Atherton, Judy Rambert, Marsha Engle, Lynn Maestro, Christie Phillips, Janet Gordon, Kathleen Bucci Bergeron and Cynthia Zahn.

And finally, thanks to all my fellow seekers who are looking to infuse your lives with peace, joy and love. And striving to live a more simple, natural, and organic lifestyle—one that's in tune with nature, and thus spirit.

FOREWORD

It's now well known that our experiences in consciousness can change the physiology of the brain. We incorporate every wisp of experience into the molecules of our body. This knowledge teaches us that we can exert powerful healing influences in our lives. As we think, so we become. If you're in a place of presence in all you do, then you change your neurochemistry. It's mind over matter. It's the power of hope and belief.

In this book, Mary Beth Janssen shares this knowledge with us in her unique and authentic voice. After years of providing high-level wellness and aesthetic services, Mary Beth understands the honor and importance of serving others from the heart. She works energetically and with great presence through the breath, through yoga, and through the senses—incorporating touch, smell, sound, visual delights, and real organic nutrition.

When we look in the mirror and we like what we see, we feel good, and our love for ourselves, others, and our environment can flow uninhibited. This awakening is the beginning of true health and harmony. The beauty we see in ourselves and around us—the aesthetic sense—is of tremendous importance determining how we feel and supporting our ability to heal. Mary Beth is a master of inspiring others on their path. She shows us that we can deeply affect our own inner and outer beauty. She encourages us to witness our thoughts and actions, making choices that give us pleasure, make us feel good, and create balance in our lives. This is not only her business and her livelihood but also her passion and her practice. Mary Beth's message has been amplified through her affiliation with Dr. Deepak Chopra, Dr. David Simon, Dr. Samuel Epstein, and the many others who have a medical and scientific grounding in the field of mind-body and holistic health.

Many people want to follow a spiritual path and create wholeness in their lives, but doing so requires consistent practice. It's through the practice that we begin to deeply feel. And it's through the feeling that endorses the knowing that a healing moment occurs. And that healing moment manifests itself as a chemical response. This intelligence becomes a frequency that settles into or occupies all chemical matter. It occupies the soil; the body, tissue, and bone structure; and the water in the environment and in our body—the matrix of life. It's part of our energetic structure. It's the sun energy and its vibration. It's the relationship between minerals, water, plants, and humans. This is the cosmic web, the interconnectedness of all life.

In this book, Mary Beth inspires us to instill these healing methods into our daily lives. Through our own practice—

whether it's personal, professional, or planetary—we can become mentors. The dynamic energy that radiates from us can affect those around us. In this way we create a collective consciousness. Ultimately, we pass it on to our children. This kind of knowingness can transform societies.

This book is a very important manual for practical living, in which our wholeness informs all of our choices. This is true sustainability. Congratulations to Mary Beth on this amazing book.

> —Horst Rechelbacher
>> Founder of Intelligent Nutrients; Aveda
>>> Corporation; HMR Art, Collectibles & Design;
>>> and the Horst Rechelbacher Foundation
>> Author of *Rejuvenation*, *Aveda Rituals*, *Alivelihood*,
>>> and *Minding Your Business: Profits That Restore
>>> the Planet*
>> Organic farmer, HMR Organic Plantation

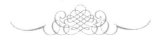

INTRODUCTION

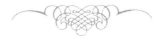

WHY PLEASURE HEALING?

"Pleasure healing," "blissful balance," and "centered wellness" are different ways of referring to a process wherein we joyfully awaken to our wholeness—and begin to heal. We set this process in motion when we weave together the layers of our being—mind, body, soul, *and* environment. This higher state of well-being—this connectedness, this heightened pleasure, this nirvana—is attainable, and in the twenty-first century, nirvana's name is "spa."

We're bombarded every day by a tremendous amount of crazy-making stress. We need a place where we can stop everything and heal, whether from traumatic experiences or from ordinary daily stress. Such healing is intrinsic to the spa universe, and this book opens wide a window into the spa's pleasure-healing sphere of influence, making it available for all of us to enjoy.

THE SPA ETHOS

The spa ethos is pure devotion to well-being, which is perhaps one reason why spas seem to be popping up like daisies worldwide. Apart from a spa, where can we find healing waters (literally and figuratively) in the desert of life? Many of us are discovering that massage, rather than Freud, can work wonders in a stressed-out life. Yoga, rather than Prozac, can open us to spirit. After all, a spa is where intimacy, sensuality, heightened consciousness (or mindfulness), and peace of mind are nurtured in an atmosphere imbued with reverential care and calm—a sacred sanctuary. A spa is where loving and appropriate touch, administered with healing hands, may be one's sole experience of touch, where compassion and nonjudgment are part of the landscape—and so instrumental in changing our *inner* landscape. Spas enrich our souls, and the sensory journey and profound healing found therein are sacred, opening us to self-knowledge, self-actualization, and enlightenment.

Spa-ing Hits the Mainstream and Goes Global

With many looking to spas for wellness, antiaging, and relaxation, "spa-ing" is the trend of the moment. Even saying the word "spa" can evoke the relaxation response! As our culture increasingly focuses on preventive health care, stress management, sustainable lifestyles, and spirituality, record numbers are turning to the spa. With spas located virtually everywhere on earth, today's spa experience can include everything from mind-body health programs and conscious-fitness programs to exotic travel and outdoor adventures. Indeed, "spa" is now accessible to the masses, because the spa aesthetic has transcended the spa environs, influencing everything from fashion, beauty, and wellness to business, travel, and leisure to architecture, home decor, and cuisine. Spa-ing *is* certifiably a cultural trend, a rejuvenating and regenerating repose from life's afflictions that balances and soothes the soul.

Sanctuaries of Spirit

As the spa universe continues to evolve, the blossoming of the "spiritual" spa is one of the most provocative concepts to date. The spiritual spa is an openhearted, celebrative community—a *satsang*, or spiritual gathering, focused on sharing creative love, healing, and passion. I've intimately experienced this kind of spa, most notably the Chopra Center for Well-Being at the La Costa Resort and Spa in Carlsbad, California, but there are many such nurturing, ecstatic, and spiritual spas. In these settings, spiritual intention turns into spiritual expression. We're encouraged to be a "yes!"—to bring out the best and brightest light in ourselves and others. The mystical, metaphysical, and cosmic-consciousness aspects of heart-centered healing connect us to our core being, so we can see ourselves as the conscious sense organs of God. Encompassing sustainability for self, home, community, and Mother Earth, the spiritual spa knows how to walk the talk, providing authenticity, which we crave now, more than ever, in our lives. The spiritual spa roots us so that we can grow and flourish. This consciousness is a calling that drives every decision, activity, service, and experience.

RELAXATION IS GOOD FOR YOU

Renewal of body, mind, and spirit—the holy grail of spa goers—is also increasingly endorsed by health care professionals, based on the integrative medical community's acknowledgment that one of the spa's greatest values is not what happens to your body during your visit but what happens to your mind that you take home with you. Spa-ing evokes the relaxation response—the opposite of the stress response. Mindfulness practices and sacred spa rituals help us break the train of stressful everyday thoughts, releasing held tension in the mind and body.

Spa Mindfulness

The spiritual spa's organic treatments, therapies, and rituals bring us into the present moment, renewing us and gently nudging the layers of our being into balance. It could be the blissful Japanese tea ceremony at Santa Fe, New Mexico's Sunrise Springs Resort Spa; the glorious organic cooking class using the on-site organic gardens at the famed Rancho La Puerta fitness resort and spa in Tecate, Mexico; a nurturing, meditative Watsu (*Water* shiatsu) session at California's renowned Harbin Hot Springs; or the sacred-loving workshops at Miraval Tucson resort and spa in Catalina, Arizona. Your pleasure-healing ritual could be the deep, healing breath your massage therapist teaches you; the mindful-eating meditation you learn from your nutritionist; or a yoga session in which you tune in to your body, listening to its various messages. It could be the body, skin, and hair care rituals provided with mindfulness by gifted hands. And there's more: from aromatherapy to labyrinth walks, mantra meditation to journal writing, laughter therapy to chakra balancing, trance dance to craniosacral therapy, Thai to Esalen massage or Reiki healing, a sweat lodge to nature vision quests. As we add these rejuvenating holistic-lifestyle approaches to our repertoire of coping skills in life's great dance, we can better elicit relaxation, which is especially valuable in helping deflect life's stressors.

The pleasure-healing activities experienced in a spa adjust your threshold for handling life's stressors with grace, aplomb, and a bit of levity thrown in for good measure. So if you haven't done so already, get thee to a spa! And certainly, having this bible in hand will serve as pure inspiration and an excellent entrée into the spa lifestyle, allowing you to infuse your life with pleasure-healing experiences as the mood strikes, whether it's your morning deep breathing and yoga stretches; a walking meditation through your neighborhood; your morning shower experienced mindfully as a cleansing ritual; your expression of gratitude for mealtime nourishment, a cup of healthy, antioxidant-steeped tea at work; or your evening aromatherapy bath.

Waking Up to Our Wakefulness

Experiences of wholeness greatly enhance our quality of life, and are always in proportion to our capacity for pleasure, delight, and joy, which is the gift of paying attention, of waking up to our wakefulness, or what some call *mindfulness*.

PLEASURE HEALING

Henry Miller wrote, "The aim of life is to live, and to live means to be aware—joyously, drunkenly, serenely, divinely aware" (1939, 76). Pleasure healing is a dynamic twenty-first century approach to *waking up* to our full human potential, higher levels of consciousness, and the resultant well-being. In a time when many of us live on the surface, pleasure healing encourages us to plunge into the depths of who we are and pay attention. When we pay exquisite attention, our energy shifts and we become the best that we can be—and have fun while we're at it—awakening and enlivening our capacity for delight.

Pleasure healing is when we engage in mindful practices and sacred rituals drawn from the spa world to nurture ourselves and elicit relaxation. As we fully engage in these experiences, deep healing ensues. Such rituals please the senses and exalt the mind and spirit, releasing a flood of feel-good chemicals into the bloodstream. There's a whole branch of science, called *psychoneuroimmunology*, that studies the interaction between the mind and body, and how this relationship affects blood chemistry. We can change our neurochemistry. Inside us is a natural pharmacy of neurochemicals that help us heal: natural antidepressants, tranquilizers, painkillers, and growth hormone, along with immunomodulators, vasodilators, and so much more. Perhaps you've heard, "Our issues are in our tissues" or "Our biography is our biology." Every thought we have creates a molecule in our bodies; this seems to be what renowned neuroscientist Dr. Candace Pert, author of the landmark book *The Molecules of Emotion*, believes. Certainly this speaks to the mind-body connection: happy thoughts create happy cells in our bodies; angry thoughts, angry cells; sad thoughts, sad cells; and so on.

Pert and Solomon Snyder, of The Johns Hopkins University, discovered the mood-enhancing, joy-inducing, pain-reducing neurohormones called endorphins (Neimark 1997). *Endorphins*, short for "endogenous morphine" (a built-in painkiller!), are released when we breathe deeply, exercise, receive a massage, make love, eat certain foods, or enjoy a host of other pleasurable activities. We can only experience the full benefit of pleasure healing when we're fully present during such experiences, which is why the theme of this book is awakening to our wholeness—our divinity, who we really are—through exquisite pleasure-healing activities enjoyed with our full attention.

From the Heart

What better place to begin on our pleasure-healing path than with the heart, our center of compassion and love? Western medicine has typically seen the heart as a pump, beating an average of seventy-two times a minute, roughly a hundred thousand times per twenty-four-hour period. In one day, your heart pumps your blood the equivalent of twelve thousand miles—the same as going almost halfway around the earth!

Each heartbeat creates an electromagnetic wave that washes over the sixty trillion cells in your body, with every cell vibrated by your heart. The heartbeat's electromagnetic frequencies can be measured up to four feet away from the body, which might be why we sense good or bad vibrations upon entering a room or situation, or why certain people have the power to cheer us up or calm us down. Good energy flows outward from such individuals, surrounding them, and they've mastered sending these healing vibrations into the universe. This is a truth that energy healers know well, and you too have this ability.

PLEASURE-HEALING RITUAL: Opening the Heart

Follow this simple practice to shift your outward flow of energy, moving you away from your fears and toward your affirmation of all that is positive.

Sit or lie down comfortably. With your eyes closed and breathing comfortably, place your palms against your chest and bring your attention to your heart center. Imagine each breath going directly into the center of your chest. Tenderly hold your breath there for a count of four. Breathing out, sense your breath moving into your palms, still placed over your heart center. With each breath, feel warmth and love being exchanged between your heart and hands. You'll begin to feel sustained warmth, tenderness, and expansion. Now slowly begin to lift your hands away, staying focused on the energetic connection between your hands and heart. Feel the warmth and love intensify. Continue making this space bigger, focusing on the feelings of love and expansion. Now imagine broadcasting these feelings outward, toward anyone you choose. Your ability to do this opens your heart to others, and importantly, you benefit as well. As we give, we receive.

After trying this, you'll easily progress to the next step. Try hugging someone lightly—heart-to-heart (your left side toward your partner's left side)—and tune in to the exchange of heart vibrations filled with love and warmth. Stay there as long as you want. This type of energy exchange, releases the "love hormone" oxytocin, relaxes and revives you, and deepens your communion with others.

Other practices for opening the heart include breathing in your own or someone else's pain and breathing out love and peace. With each breath, inhale the pain, and then exhale love. You can also radiate light by imagining a brilliant light in your heart center that shines upon everyone and everything. When you experience a conflict or problem, think of this bright light as a spotlight. Keep broadening the area upon which your spotlight shines, until finally it illuminates the conflict. Look closely to see what this conflict can teach you, and then be thankful for this learning experience.

Congratulations! This first pleasure-healing ritual shows you that the heart is one flexible muscle that can be stretched to make room for so much loving-kindness.

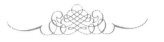

CHAPTER 1

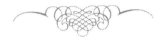

EMBRACING MINDFULNESS

When Buddha was asked, "What do you and your disciples practice?" he answered, "We sit, we walk, we eat." Perplexed, the questioner inquired, "Doesn't everyone sit, walk, and eat?" "Yes," replied Buddha, "but when we sit, we know we are sitting. When we walk, we know we are walking. When we eat, we know we are eating." This is the essence of mindfulness in our lives—the nonjudgmental awareness, or "witnessing," of the moment and our place in it, also referred to as "paying attention on purpose." Heaven is indeed here on earth in the myriad ways we devote our spirits to the minutiae of our daily lives. By integrating the two worlds, we find wholeness. When exquisitely mindful, we become extremely aware of the spiritual nature of the material world. More tuned-in, we begin to see spirit everywhere and in everything. In this state of being, we seek the spiritual root of any problem and channel our energy to heal it. It's all inside; if you're ready to do this work, spirit awaits you.

Whether you're eating a meal, washing dishes, brushing your teeth, making love, sitting in a traffic jam, or caring for an ailing loved one, be mindful of every nuance of the experience. Become the witness, consciously observing spirit. Be present in this moment, right here, right now. Watch yourself reading these words and reflecting on them.

Stop resisting life; let moments arise as they are, without labeling them. When you're not mindful, life is less satisfying; you're usually somewhere else, striving for what's missing, but in fact, *you're* what's missing. Imagine being with a group of friends at a beautiful sunset. Everyone except you drinks in the glorious view. Rather than enjoy the sunset, you let the moment's richness pass you by. In a balanced life, mindfulness prevents the moments that are the fabric of our lives from going by in a blur. Rather, we learn to savor them, much the way we did as children, when the days seemed long.

When you're fully present as each moment unfolds, your life changes dramatically, with the potential to become vibrant and electrifying beyond compare. We see the fullness of what *is*, rather than what's lacking. Now let's be honest; if we reflect on it, any one of us could find a number of annoyances in our daily lives. It's how you allow them to affect you that matters. When you're fully present, accepting and living a life of joy, you can shrug or laugh them off. Individuals at a crossroads see them as a blueprint for change, whereas those who are out of touch with spirit, depressed, or anxious just skid on them into a ditch. Being fully present conveys the knowledge to make choices about stressful situations. And importantly, if the problem can't be solved, you can change your perception or learn better coping skills. Yes, mindfulness encourages you to consciously work with your own stress, pain, illness, and everyday challenges instead of simply "stuffing" them.

We may be distracted by the persistent needs of the ego: the need for power, control, and approval. Spirit doesn't have any of these needs. Spirit just *is*, right now, in this moment. This is the real you. Mindfulness connects you to spirit, and when it does, you make the most life-affirming choices for yourself rather than those from learned habits or physical needs. For example, consider how you wake up. Do you bolt out of bed and stumble to the shower, barely aware of the time, date, or century? To witness your own morning and nurture your life-force energy, wake up slowly. Make awakening a delightful ritual. Do a bit of yoga (even in bed!), enjoy a moment of meditation, practice self-massage, step in the shower, and become one with the water. As you move through your day, greet people in a nonjudgmental and compassionate way. "Compassion" is a word you'll see throughout this book. Compassion is a practice—and the ultimate sign of emotional maturity. In yoga we speak of *ahimsa*, or noninjury, as one of the most important practices for living joyfully and developing universal love. Ahimsa is refraining from causing pain to any living creature. So it is also with compassion, which calls upon us to be kind from the awareness that everyone carries some form of burden.

One of my mentors, Deepak Chopra, has said in many of his seminars, "We're all doing the best we can from the level of consciousness we're in." Everyone's level of consciousness differs depending on life circumstances. When you try to understand where someone is coming from, you automatically become less judgmental. As you become less judgmental, you become more tolerant; when more tolerant, you're better able to forgive. And when you can forgive, you have the capacity to love unconditionally. Compassion creates a remarkable chain of positive energy that results in the most radiant well-being possible.

PLEASURE-HEALING RITUAL: Housecleaning

To celebrate life in such a broad, unprejudiced manner, many of us may need to consider a little emotional cleansing and a few attitude changes. It's important to understand that much of our stress is relative to our perception of a given situation. When you learn how to change your perception of, or emotional attitude toward, stressful situations, you remove their ability to negatively affect you. I'm not suggesting that you try to bypass painful or uncomfortable feelings; we need to fully sit with these emotions and listen to them. But it's how we process them that truly matters.

To begin the cleansing process, try observing your emotions. Begin simply, by looking at one emotion that's at the top of your mind today. Commit to taking full responsibility for the emotion. It's quite easy to place the blame elsewhere for our anger, sadness, or bitterness, when these are, in fact, our feelings; we create them as readily as we diffuse them. Identify the sensations that the emotion creates in your body. Verbalize or write down how the emotion makes you feel. What can this emotion teach you about yourself? What needs do you have that are unmet? Have the intention to clearly define this, and work toward resolving the unmet need. Now release the emotion and consciously celebrate this release. The emotion no longer controls you, but you control it! If this technique seems overwhelming, ask a friend or loved one for support, or consider getting professional help. Talking to someone who is removed from your stressful situation can bring tremendous relief, renewal, and even rebirth.

PLEASURE-HEALING RITUAL: Mindfulness

Though mindfulness takes practice, as with forming any new habit (usually thirty days), it can become second nature. "Witness" your thoughts from the time you get up in the morning until you go to bed at night. Narrate your day to yourself, "Good morning, self," and do so with great interest and enthusiasm.

Cultivate the practice of noticing what you habitually pay attention to and what you ignore. To paraphrase Jesus, "Where your attention is, there will your heart be also." If you reflect on what you pay attention to throughout the day, what does this say about you? What priority would love and soulful connection with others have in the arc of your day? Would you like to change your investments in attention, time, and concern?

MINDFULNESS TRIGGERS CAN HELP

Mindfulness triggers remind you to relax and be at peace, more spontaneous and free. Choose a word, phrase, or activity to trigger mindfulness if your attention has lapsed or floated off into the ether. Continually returning to awareness allows your daily activities and your life to take on a meditative quality. You can perform any action with awareness, even pouring a glass of water, hanging up your phone, or turning off your computer. Every time you do even the smallest action, take a deep breath, noticing how your muscles relax. Repeating as necessary will make it easier to have a relaxed state of being. I encourage my students to place sticky notes with such words as "breathe!" "relax!" or "smile!" wherever they'll see them on a regular basis: on the bathroom mirror or the computer, in the car, and so on. You can also sketch, paint, or embroider your word; frame it; and place it by your bed, on the bathroom wall, or by your work area (it's also a nice gift idea). You can mentally use a phrase or image to shift your awareness, such as *Be Here Now*, the name of the classic book by Ram Dass (also known as *Remember, Be Here Now*).

Look for transitions during your day to cultivate mindfulness, such as making a phone call, walking through a doorway, getting in your car, picking up the mail, taking a meal, or taking your first sip of tea. For instance, instead of habitually grabbing the phone when it rings, take a moment to roll your shoulders down away from your ears, take a deep breath, and smile before picking up the phone. This simple process can be amazingly transformative. Your calm energy and friendly smile will travel across the phone lines!

You can also take a moment to feel the beating of your heart. Its rhythm is your rhythm. If you rush ahead of your heart's rhythm, chances are that you'll miss much of what's really important in your life. Bring your attention to your heartbeat and take several deep, cleansing breaths.

Your daily ablutions can also be mindfulness rituals. When taking a shower, step inside, be fully present with the core of your being, and breathe deeply. Face the shower and feel it rain on your skin; really feel the water on your skin. Engage all your senses with the feel and sound of the water, and the smell of your body wash or shampoo. Imagine all tension streaming from your skin's surface and down the drain. Being fully present during any and all personal care rituals is a delightful way to begin or end your day. This is truly "conscious" care.

MAKING THE CONNECTION

A variety of daily practices can bring exquisite mindfulness of the life-force energy that permeates and surrounds all of creation. Witness everything you do. Observe yourself reading this sentence right now. "Be here now." When you eat, really taste your food. When you're with someone, really be with that person. Look into his or her eyes and see the soul residing there. In bed tonight, rise above your body and observe yourself shifting from wakefulness to sleep.

Commit to practicing healing breath, meditation, positive affirmations, visualization, and a mindful physical activity, such as yoga or tai chi. Each practice hones our sensitivity to mindfulness, allowing our sprit to soar into uncharted waters—and the realm of infinite possibilities.

Get lost in organic and sacred rituals. Burn your favorite incense or candle, and connect with the aroma, color, and movement of the embers. Play enchanting music, hearing each individual note as well as the harmony. Read poetry aloud and listen to the rhyme and texture of the words.

Enjoy the sensual feast inherent in nature. See the details in the clouds, trees, rocks, and water. See the universe in a leaf. See divinity in a blade of grass or the petals of a flower. Feel the sun on your face and the wind in your hair. Listen to nature's primordial sounds. Look for the man in the moon.

Create beauty. Expand your creativity where you've not ventured before. Sketch, paint, mold clay, or make a mosaic or ornament. Get lost in the process. Whatever you create exemplifies organic beauty.

Construct an altar at home or work. Whether it's on a windowsill or a huge oak table, place things that have meaning for you: a loved one's photo, a lock of hair, a feather, a rosary, or a gem. This altar will gently remind you of spirit's presence, eliciting tranquility and centeredness.

Let your soul write. Keep a journal each and every day. Write down whatever's on your mind, without editing or censoring. You'll experience so many insights.

Cultivate peace in a garden, whether in an acre out back or a terra-cotta pot on your veranda. Visualize how it will look after your TLC, and then set out to bring this beauty home. See your garden as a metaphor for your inner garden, which you tend by planting, feeding, weeding, and harvesting.

Spend a day indulging in beautifying rituals. Visit a spa and let a cadre of pros treat you to an experience of sheer bliss. Or invite a friend over and perform beautifying rituals on each other.

Tune-in to the cosmic rhythms, the calendar of the soul. Honor the sun, moon, and stars. Celebrate the seasons, whether it's spring's blossoms bursting open and a resurgence of energy everywhere or winter's retreat deep into the earth for a season of introspection. Both are great metaphors to feast on.

Honor significant stages in your life and those of your loved ones. This may mean something as seemingly small as cutting out an hour of television every night to make quiet time to meditate, or it may be huge events, such as giving birth, getting married, or losing a loved one. Honor them all!

PLEASURE-HEALING RITUAL: Beginner's Mind

Marcel Proust said, "The real voyage of discovery consists not in seeking new landscapes but in having new eyes." This beautifully expresses the Buddhist practice of *beginner's mind*, a mind-set that allows us to appreciate old information with "new eyes," setting aside the know-it-all, seen-it-all, done-it-all mind-set that diminishes enthusiasm and undervalues the tried and true. Beginner's mind offers innocence, wonderment, and openness to possibility, encouraging us to take everything we know—opinions, preconceived notions, and even cherished beliefs—and put them away for a while. (Don't worry; they'll be there when you get back!) It also encourages you to say, "I don't know" (even if you think you know). "I know" prevents us from understanding the present moment's mysteries, and keeps us living in the past; we close ourselves off to the surprises or discoveries that give life zest.

Just throw up your hands and say, "I don't know!" Not knowing is a wonderful state to be in, so innocent and liberating. Beginner's mind knows that in the most familiar circumstances are riches to be unearthed. You think you know your husband? How about your children? How about your mom? How about your boss? There's always much more there to discover. You can glance along the surface or really delve in deep, where infinite possibilities reside. Beginner's mind allows you to see your world anew every day so that, in every moment, old information can bring fresh insights.

Take one day at a time in developing beginner's mind. Watch when the inner know-it-all rears its ugly head, and bring your attention back to spirit. Meditation fosters a beginner's mind, inspires us, and jump-starts positive change, while helping to de-emphasize the programming that replays over and over in our minds, driving our unconscious behavior.

Speaking of positivity, in the morning, look in the mirror and tell yourself, "Every day, in every way, I'm getting better and better" or "Today's a new day, and I can choose a different path." And no matter what happens, set your intention to receive value from your experiences. Energy follows intention.

PLEASURE-HEALING RITUAL: Intentionality

If you want to change some aspect of your life, direct your mind toward a goal, or manifest your dreams, start by setting an intention—making the deliberate decision to create something or intend that something happen. Intentions aren't fleeting thoughts or wishes, but rather, they're like sacred rocket fuel, turning your good but half-baked ideas into brilliant, fully formed bullet points. They allow you to visualize and clarify what matters most to you. Intentions help you "jack up" your commitment level, whatever the undertaking, be it losing weight; exercising; meditating daily;

being kind; learning something new; or fulfilling your dharma, or life's purpose. You can set an intention anytime, anywhere. It's powerful to focus your awareness on an intention before beginning contemplative practice. Then you'll operate from a place of fluidity and calm, where intuition, intelligence, and sensory perception are heightened.

Follow up on your intention by taking action that supports it. All this dynamic energy then flows in the same direction. If you set an intention but the energy of your action flows in a different direction, a positive outcome is less likely. Let's look at an example: if you intend to improve your relationship with your significant other and your follow-up actions are to have meaningful conversation, check in with phone calls or e-mail during the day, or give a shoulder rub, it's highly probable your relationship will improve. However, if your actions oppose your intent—for example, you come home late without phoning or explaining, verbally abuse your partner, or ignore him or her—then the opposing energies will *cause* friction and stress. Setting an intention and directing your energy toward the desired outcome through your actions will surely balance your life and manifest your desires.

Use the mantra, "Energy follows intention," for whatever changes you seek in your life. Meditate on your intention or write it down, and then consider potential follow-up actions. Do the energies of the actions flow in the same direction as your intention? Many give lip service to changing, but their actions don't match their intentions; take New Year's resolutions, for example! We get frustrated with the process of change (what I call "self-improvement fatigue" or "boredom") or feel we've failed again. The truth is that our actions aren't aligned with our intentions. Either the action or the intention needs to change.

The intention statement helps align your actions with your inner values. The words you use to verbalize your intention amplify the power of thought, creating an energetic imprint. Our nervous system responds to an intention statement clearly focused on the intent. To say "I intend to do whatever it takes to feel relaxed and happy today" is very clear and focused on how your actions can support your well-being. This works better than saying "I hope to _____," where you almost give yourself permission to come short of your goal, or "I want to _____," where you're too attached to a method of achieving it. Both are a bit wishy-washy! Play around with these statements for what you want to create in your life, and you'll experience the difference. A properly constructed intention statement puts your attention on the ever-present now in the constantly changing flow of life.

VISUALIZATION AND POSITIVE AFFIRMATIONS

Visualization and positive affirmations are powerful tools for invoking the relaxation response, and when used in tandem with mindfulness, beginner's mind, and intentionality, they influence you to become the "witness," the dreamer, the creator, the lover—inspiring and opening you to the infinite possibilities on this earthly plane. Together, they encourage you to choose your values, dreams, and goals; see and positively sense your purpose in being here; and go forward to plan, enact, and create a life of meaning and enjoyment. This is the path to fulfilling your dharma, your life's purpose.

Visualization is a powerful practice you can use anytime to form desirable images in your mind's eye. See yourself doing exactly what you want to do, such as eating an ice-cream cone, walking along the beach, or playing with a child. Try to see whatever makes you happy. Little by little, zoom your image outward until you engage all five senses in this imagery. When you feel comfortable with this part of the exercise, you're ready for the tough stuff. Now envision fulfilling deep desires or goals. Place your intention and attention where you want your consciousness to be. Think as big as you want!

But be careful what you wish for! Visualization is a powerful tool for taking action, and wishes can come true. Visualizing from the heart can evoke relaxation and, further, help you manifest exquisite well-being, harmonious relationships, the perfect job, and, when collectively done, even world peace.

Visualization is sometimes called "mental rehearsal." Sports physiologists teach Olympic athletes to envision every nuance of the next day's performance. Physicians teach patients to envision health. Lance Armstrong not only used visualization to win the Tour de France but also to fight off testicular cancer. Before giving presentations to large audiences, I "see" myself perform to the best of my ability.

PLEASURE-HEALING RITUAL: All Aboard for Shangri-la!

See yourself in a beautiful scene at a relaxing place. It can be a familiar place full of memories or somewhere you've never been. Close your eyes and imagine the scene as if you were watching a movie screen—in living color! In your mind's eye, become intimate with every nuance of this place. Use all your senses. Experience the colors, aromas, textures, and sounds. Feel the movement of air. If you're on the beach, feel the saltwater mist on your skin. If you're drinking an exotic fruit drink, taste the natural sweetness of this nectar. Breathe deeply as you continue visualizing for five to ten minutes. Now take the time to think about what you've seen. If the experience seemed real, in going from profound relaxation to exhilaration, your mind-body physiology will react as if it *were* real.

You'll find this technique powerful for programming your subconscious to enhance your sense of well-being. Visualize yourself in loving relationships or experiencing joy and lightheartedness. Visualize your body as strong and toned, your skin as smooth and glowing. Visualize your eyes as vibrant, clear, and dazzling. You may just manifest what you visualize!

Visualization can also cut through our mental chatter to transform behavior or thought patterns. The more you practice, the better you get at this. That beautiful, imaginary scene could be your destination when you're facing a perplexing challenge. Visualize yourself in your relaxing place, perhaps sitting against a tree or lying on the beach, imagining a solution to your problem. Let yourself see the desired outcome to any challenge. You might see how to mend a relationship rift, present a new idea, meet someone for the first time with grace and calm, optimally get your work done, manage stress, or overcome fear. You can focus on more-practical, serenity-inducing matters, such as sitting with a heavenly fragranced conditioning treatment on your hair and visualizing the results. Or see yourself on your morning walk, with your body and mind getting healthier, stronger, and more vital. Practice often. Visualization is powerful for programming your subconscious to follow a desired path.

POSITIVE AFFIRMATIONS: BEHOLD THE BEAUTY WITHIN

Do you know how beautiful you are? Yes, you! You're beautiful beyond compare. Affirm this to yourself ten times right here and now. I'll wait.

Okay, now that you're back, think about how you felt as you affirmed your beauty. Did you feel a spark of power? What if you used that spark to ignite filling your whole life with beauty, truth, and goodness? Imagine this tiny spark spiraling outward, casting a radiant glow upon everything and every person you see. Can you picture how glorious it would be to see all of life in this beautiful light of transformation? Once you achieve this, you'll find more to celebrate and less to criticize. Now, imagine how those around you—family, friends, and business associates—will feel as they interact with you. How do you think they'll react to you as a person who sees beauty in the entire world and everyone in it? This brings to mind words attributed to Mahatma Gandhi: "We must become the change we want to see." The residual effects of your self-realized beauty are enormous. Together we're exploring ways to turn your spark into a radiant blaze.

Let's ignite that spark, shall we? But first, let's dwell some more on how beautiful you are! Affirm it. Spend the next few moments thinking about, appreciating, and writing down all that you find beautiful in yourself and your life. Let the words flow unedited.

What would I write? Oh, something like this: I appreciate my curly hair and long legs; my nonjudgmental nature; my athletic ability; my deep compassion for humanity and all of creation; my wonderful husband; my cherished family; my wonderful friends and dear clients; my adorable pet companions; the air that I breathe; the nutritious food that I eat; pure water to drink; toilets that flush; my meditation and yoga practice; having enough money to pay the bills; the first tomatoes out of the garden; my glorious, scarlet-red poppies opening for their brief spring fling; and Friday-night martinis.

Now, get out your notebook or journal and try it yourself. What beauty do you appreciate in your life?

Abe Lincoln said, "Most folks are as happy as they make up their minds to be." We can all embrace bliss, joy, happiness, optimism, and positivity as long as it's a life goal. Who doesn't want to be happy? According to a survey of 6,500 American women, 95 percent said that happiness was more important to them than power, wealth, or even beauty. We all have our down days, but a basic capacity for bliss is the foundation for overcoming even the most trying obstacles. This means enjoying a steady diet of simple pleasures rather than waiting for that big pie in the sky. Our inner lives, relationships, and careers are the areas in our personal landscapes most likely to send us sinking into a well of self-pity or soaring into a cloud of self-satisfaction. Getting a grip on these areas gives us the ability to experience the essence of true joy. So how about you? Are you for floating in a sea of serenity or watching from the shore in fear of riding that big wave of bliss?

BE THE OPTIMIST

Pleasure healing is about holistic thinking. One attitude that beautifully supports holistic thinking is optimism, our ability to see the best in everyone and everything. It gives us the perceptiveness to see a beautiful and good world and to learn and grow from all that we experience, positive or negative.

Here's an example: Say something's been stolen from you. Naturally, this feels like a violation. In many respects, it is, but if you shift your perception to detachment, you may be able to see that whoever took this thing must have needed it more than you! Eliciting this type of energy can prevent feelings of grief, sadness, or victimization. This is not to belittle that something was stolen from you or deny that you deserve to feel a moment of anger, but quickly getting over it and focusing on a feeling of optimism will get you through the situation more quickly so that you come out of it with your mind-body health in a much better place, if not totally unscathed.

Beyond enjoying emotional benefits, optimists have higher levels of natural killer cell activity, so they tend to be more capable of fighting disease. Optimists also have lower levels of the stress hormone cortisol (Arnot 2000). Optimism develops tremendous resiliency, the ability to take what life hands you and get through it, get over it, and get on with it. It's the ability to be challenged without breaking down.

What makes a person resilient? The ability to feel connected to others. Resilient people tend to be self-reliant, flexible, and capable of nurturing personal relationships. These people are also able to learn from bad events rather than feel like a victim.

We all experience misfortunes and losses; it's part of our destiny. Yet, it's exactly these setbacks that can serve to strengthen our will. Be the optimist. Allow yourself to bounce back. Don't stop enjoying the wonder and miracle of life.

PLEASURE-HEALING RITUAL: Spread Your Wings and Fly

Having affirmed how truly beautiful you are, let's see how far we can take this positive self-talk. For the next twenty-four hours, shower yourself with positive affirmations. Having trouble getting started? Try one of these affirmations:

- Each day is a new beginning, a fresh start.
- I'm alive and filled with vitality.
- I'm so glad to be me!
- Every day, I appreciate who I am and what I have.
- My positive way of thinking is changing my world.

- I have the courage to be myself without fear or apology.
- I'm learning and growing by dropping old prejudices.
- My life is as happy and full as possible without my harming myself, others, or the planet.
- We're all in this big soup together, loving, learning, and living to our fullest capacity.

Now put pencil to paper and write your own affirmations. However you choose to express an affirmation, clearly celebrate it. Before meditating in the morning, speak the words as a form of grace. Smile and relish them as you speak! Sing the affirmation in verse if you'd like. Ultimately you'll program your subconscious to expect great things every day.

THE COSMIC DANCE

There's a beautiful ancient saying: "If you want to know what your experiences were like in the past, look at your body today; and if you want to know what your body will look like in the future, look at your experiences today." If you're unhappy with how your mind-body physiology fares, you can change it through your experiences. The human body isn't merely static matter but, rather, vibrating energy. At the deepest level of being, we're subatomic particles whirling around at lightning speed through vast open space, on the verge of becoming matter. And matter is on the verge of becoming energy. This fluctuation of energy and matter is life's cosmic dance. Seven million red blood cells blink in and out of existence in your body every second. Your pancreas regenerates every twenty-four hours, your stomach lining every three days, your white blood cells every ten days, your brain protein every month, your liver every six weeks. You shed a hundred thousand skin cells every minute! Your body will be different by the time you finish reading this sentence than when you started. Successfully performing this renewal process requires nourishment in the form of optimal thought, food, and activity. If changing our experiences benefits our mind-body physiology, let's do it! Each of us has the power to make choices that create balance and harmony in our lives. The good news is that changing our experiences sometimes means little more than changing our *perceptions* of those experiences.

To connect with these amazing discoveries, you may have to release fears that have been holding you back and preventing you from accepting something new. All there is in life is either love or fear. Yet fear can be strong, and letting go is often a gradual process.

To let go of fear, it helps to look more closely at *why* certain things scare you into numbness or tunnel vision. Many common fears stem from a general fear of change. Begin here, asking yourself, "What is it about change that scares me?" Do any of the following responses hit home?

Fear of failure: Accepting change means dealing with something new, and any time we approach the unfamiliar, there's a possibility that we won't get it right the first time.

Fear of commitment: With change comes the unknown, and committing to the unknown might lead to disappointment.

Fear of disapproval: If we embrace change and then fail to produce tried-and-true results, we might disappoint others and have to deal with their disapproval.

Fear of success: Success is a wonderful thing, but it often brings with it added responsibilities, expectations, and goals.

Life-Force Energy

Tapping into our energy source can manifest all our desires and help us learn to work through change positively; fears be damned! We have the power to become the mystic, sage, or shaman, playing fearlessly in this extremely fluid and changeable world. It all begins when we shift our consciousness toward our higher good and away from the possible missteps along the way.

Let's put a positive spin on the fears listed earlier and shift our focus to our higher consciousness through positive affirmations:

- I love experimentation, and I will use this creative drive to control my fear of failure.

- I love my ability to break larger goals into achievable steps, and I will use this tactic to conquer my fear of commitment.

- I love myself, and I will use this self-appreciation to conquer my fear of disapproval.

- I love to celebrate life, and I will use this joyous energy to control my fear of success.

Now you give it a try: (1) open your notebook or journal and list four reasons why you routinely fear or resist change. (2) Now view these fears through a different lens, that of higher consciousness. How can each fear be redefined through a positive affirmation about yourself?

GOOD MEDICINE

Remember this one truth: you are a healer. Your capacity for healing knows no bounds. Your creativity, actions, attitude, manner of speech, behavior, touch, words, and—yes—love all have the potential to heal. This magnificent power begins with the care you give yourself. Take any fears you have about change and turn them around until you become focused on all the good and healthy elements inherent in change. Once you harness the ability to heal your own fears, then you can begin to open your heart, sending love and kindness out to others. Our lives are about loving communion with others. We have the power to bring good medicine to everyone we touch—beginning with ourselves. It's our dharma, our purpose in life.

CHAPTER 2

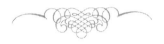

TRANSFORMING STRESS INTO BALANCE

Health and disease don't just happen to us. They are active processes issuing from inner harmony or disharmony, profoundly affected by our states of consciousness, our ability or inability to flow with experience.

—MARILYN FERGUSON

In his book, *Managing Stress*, Brian Luke Seaward defines stress as the *inability to cope* with a real or imagined threat to our well-being, which results in a series of responses and adaptations by our minds and bodies (Seaward 1997, 5). I stress "inability to cope," because having healthy coping strategies to deflect the stressors we're faced with—whether real or imagined—is essential to our well-being. We're all going to be faced with traumas, tragedies, and shocks over our lifetimes. It's how we cope with these stressors that determines our ability to realize exquisite wholeness and go the distance.

Some say that our bodies have become so acclimated to change that now we can speed up but can't slow down. Change continues in overdrive. Many changes are considered progress, but some seem downright regressive. Even those viewed as improvements can come at a price, for even progress can bring deep-rooted insecurities due to globalization and political and sociocultural influences. There's no place to hide from these influences, because the media feeds us a daily diet of worldwide disaster. Now add in the personal stressors we face. Such constant exposure to life's challenges and frailties can cause overwhelming stress—if we don't have coping mechanisms in place.

IDENTIFYING STRESSORS

Many healers today believe that we're disconnected from our deepest, truest selves, distracted and overwhelmed by the sheer speed of life. Wherever we turn, we're told how we should look, act, feel, and be. We're dancing as fast as we can to accommodate society's standards. Consequently we're losing our balance and tripping over every little fad. Sadly, as we lose contact with our inner selves, we create a breeding ground for stress. We're well on our way toward managing stress and finding true healing with the practices we've explored thus far—but there's so much more.

We need to remember how to lighten up. Take laughter, for instance. Laughter is a huge step toward enlightenment. It's also "carbonated holiness," according to the theology of one of my favorite writers, Anne Lamott. When was the last time you laughed so hard that tears rolled down your cheeks and your belly muscles ached? Laughter truly is the shortest distance between two people; and it's the number one personality trait we look for in a romantic partner! But with the stressors we face, it's easy to squelch the belly laughs. Voltaire said, "God is a comedian playing to an audience too afraid to laugh." Make a concerted effort to bring the healing peals of laughter into your life. Be a human sunbeam amid the chaos. At the very least, smile. A smile and a kind word may very well be one of the best tools to diffuse tension, or lift your or another's spirits.

PLEASURE-HEALING RITUAL: Laughter Therapy

To offset stress, the Association for Applied and Therapeutic Humor recommends laughter as an antidote. Research shows that laughter reduces stress hormones and has definite healing properties (Berk 1996). It triggers the release of endorphins into the bloodstream, improving mood and reducing pain, as well as elevates brain awareness and fends off disease by activating immunological cells.

Did you know children laugh on average four hundred times a day, while adults only experience fifteen such chuckles in a typical day (Gilda's Club Chicago 2003)? So protect and hold dear your child within. Generally, children haven't yet had time to let their inner censor take over, that mighty reflex that frowns on new ideas, prohibits unbridled laughter, forbids the heartfelt tear, and scoffs at business-*not*-as-usual.

To bring more laughter into your life:

- Share the humor. When you hear or read something that tickles your funny bone, pass it on and laugh all over again.

- Choose your friends carefully. Those who make you laugh are a treasure. Distance yourself from those who are whiners or perpetually put out a doom-and-gloom vibe.

- Take up a new interest, preferably with someone you like. Rudimentary attempts at anything new can bring on hysterics, if you let them. Just remember, don't take yourself too seriously.

- Poke fun at yourself—or anything for that matter. Look for life's many absurdities. If you're not naturally funny, just concentrate on having fun! The laughs will come.

- Keep funny movies on hand or rent them, and visit one of the many websites devoted to all things humorous. Read funny articles and jokes, or buy a humorous CD or book.

- Look into joining or starting a local laughter club. Members engage in laughing exercises that flow into spontaneous laughter. I personally belong to one and can vouch for the incredible feeling of well-being, camaraderie, and fun they conjure! Check out www .worldlaughtertour.com or www.laughteryoga.org.

THE STRESS RESPONSE

Stress is a normal part of life and is a good thing, to a point. *Eustress* is when we channel our energy to see the glass half full and perform at our optimal best. Eustress provides the zest that kick-starts motivation and runs a positive, enthusiastic mental soundtrack. Such manageable stress gives us uncommon strength and fortitude to achieve goals and face a challenge or perceived threat.

Stress results from the body's instinct to defend itself from physical, mental, emotional, and environmental stressors, whether real or imagined. This includes the "fight-or-flight" response, which helps in emergencies, such as getting out of the way of a speeding car. But stress causes substantial harm if allowed to hum along unabated in response to life's daily challenges and changes. The resulting *distress* is responsible for a wide range of chronic and acute *dis*-ease. Our bodies respond to stress by making stress hormones (adrenaline, cortisol, and other corticosteroids) that help us respond as needed in extreme situations. But if we make too many of these hormones, over time they wear us down.

Uncontrolled stress blocks the flow of life-force energy, negatively affecting the central nervous system and blood chemistry, along with cardiovascular, endocrine, respiratory, gastrointestinal, and immune system functions. It can exhaust the adrenal glands, impair memory, raise blood pressure, inhibit the immune system's ability to fight infection, raise blood-sugar levels, destabilize insulin levels, promote musculoskeletal problems, and even destroy brain cells. It also creates an overabundance of free radicals, which are at the core of oxidation of bodily tissue and aging. Over time, stress *can* kill.

Our creativity, joie de vivre, and love for our fellow human beings all suffer when we're in the throes of stress. Stress can transform us from calm, compassionate, joyful human beings into fiery "rageaholics," fearful scaredy-cats, or depressed and moody couch potatoes.

COMING OUT OF STRESS AND INTO BALANCE

We're the sum of what we think, feel, and do. These combined activities make up our health profile. Regularly indulging in stress-inducing behaviors doesn't honor our wholeness, so disharmony sets in. If we consistently function on high-speed fast-forward, skip meals, eat junk foods, smoke, take drugs, forego exercise, sleep poorly, lack direction and focus, are pessimistic, have little love in our lives, and lack spiritual connection, we're placing ourselves at risk for a catastrophic illness.

If we ground ourselves and come from a place of balance, our interactions will be from the highest level of consciousness. Some profound and soulful energy is transmitted during such encounters. Creating these experiences in consciousness dramatically enhances calmness, compassion, enthusiasm, joy, creativity, and intuition.

Staying Centered

Pascal said, "There is pleasure in being in a ship beaten about by a storm when we are sure that it will not founder." Centered in self, you won't founder when life's stressors brew around you. In this mind-numbing, attention-deficit world, we can't totally eradicate toxic stress from our lives. Yet we can learn to greatly reduce and manage stressors by changing how we *perceive and respond* to them. Stress can only harm your health *if* you let it.

Yes, this is a tall order, but affirm and know that you're in control of your life. You'll get to this place of "centeredness" and conscious witnessing of what you're doing in any given moment through daily contemplative practice, where you tune in to who's at the core of your being. There's a beautiful, ancient saying: "In a pure mind, there is constant awareness of Self. Where there is constant awareness of Self, freedom ends bondage, and joy ends sorrow."

When you can control your *reaction* to potentially stressful situations, you have the power to conquer stress. Being centered in Self gives you power. The greatest antidote for stress is fully awakening to your true nature and its guidance for making life-affirming choices.

Assess Your Stress

So ask yourself, do you have a handle on the stress in your own sphere of influence? Your day may involve a tightly packed schedule and interaction with various personality types and energies, with your brainpower and creativity called upon to make many decisions using intuition and discernment. Maybe you also move your body through a wide range of postures and positions (or maybe not move much at all!) and experience poor nutrition, environmental toxicity, and compromised sleep, all of which can have a dramatic impact on your mind-body physiology and energy levels—if you *let* them.

Life holds the potential for layer upon layer of stressors: the dance of relationships, paying bills, running a household, losing loved ones, caring for children or aging parents, illnesses, the news of war and mayhem, deepening environmental degradation, and most certainly the incredible time crunch to try to fit it all in! Just writing all of this starts my stress hormones flowing! But a few shoulder-releasing yoga asanas (postures), and ten deep diaphragmatic breaths later, I'm cool as a cucumber, one with the universe, *and* have stopped the damaging flow of stress hormones in their tracks.

The following short list can help you to check your stress levels. Do you:

- Often feel tired and lack energy?

- Have a problem controlling your emotions and easily become anxious, agitated, or unhappy, even when faced with minor problems?

- Have problems falling or staying asleep?

- Keep rehashing what you should've, could've, or would've done instead of moving onward?

- Often have the feeling that something dreadful might happen?

- Often have trouble sitting still or concentrating?

- Feel pain in your chest, a racing heart, or shortness of breath?

- Regularly experience gastrointestinal upsets, including heartburn, constipation, or diarrhea?

- Often have musculoskeletal pain, especially in the back, neck, and shoulders?

- Have frequent headaches?

- Feel nervous or sweat a lot?

- Smoke or drink alcohol excessively?

If you answered yes to even a few of these questions, take special care to integrate as many of the rituals in this book as you can to reduce your stress.

COPING POSITIVELY

Contemplative practices and sensory-modulation techniques can dramatically alter our consciousness and shift our energy to a higher vibrational realm, where transformation and great healing can take place.

We bring balance into our lives through our choices. Many healthy choices are as simple as creating a daily routine that promotes stability, which is a wonderfully soothing mechanism whenever everything else is chaotic. A routine gives you time and space to connect mind, body, and spirit. What's nice is that this step toward balance doesn't come in a bottle, is accessible to everyone, and costs nothing.

PLEASURE-HEALING RITUAL: Let Your Soul Write

A journal is a personal record of your deepest thoughts, feelings, attitudes, perceptions, and behaviors. When you've written honestly, your journal can bring you face to face with the naked truth of yourself. Journal-keeping is simply one of the best self-awareness tools—and one of my favorite consciousness-raising experiences. It can help you see where patterns of dissonance or chaos occur in your life, and allow you to reflect on and be grateful for the joys life brings.

Writing down whatever's on your mind—from the most mundane to the most bizarre thoughts, and everything in between—will prove tremendously cathartic for your soul, allowing you to clear out the gunk, vent your feelings, and make some important self-discoveries along the way. For instance, you'll probably spot repetitive thoughts; these point to areas in your life that need extra attention. Try to write a few passages every day.

It's especially helpful to have your journal handy when you're struggling with a particular issue. Write a few words about what's going on. Note your feelings and the sensations these feelings create in your body and mind. If you're in the midst of a difficult experience, talk it through with just you and your journal. And

41

certainly, if you experience any form of fulfillment, exhilaration, love, or gratitude, note this as well. Acknowledging good feelings allows you to more readily see and feel the grace around you, and thus become an expression of this love and grace. You're writing your life's story in your journal's pages, and the process of writing brings your experiences fully into your consciousness.

PLEASURE-HEALING RITUAL: Progressive Relaxation

It's said that we have sixty thousand thoughts a day, and fifty-nine thousand of them are reruns from yesterday! That's a lot of chatter! In Eastern philosophy this replaying is called "monkey mind." Following is a classic yet simple practice for bringing you back into your body and out of your monkey mind quicker than you can say "relax."

1. Sit or lie in a comfortable position. Close your eyes and rhythmically breathe in and out.

2. Begin at the crown of your head. Notice any tension in your scalp, and give yourself permission to let it go. Move onward to the forehead and face, doing the same. Let your shoulders melt down away from your ears, and release your jaw. Remember to soften the "inner" body.

3. Progressively move your attention from the top of your head to the tips of your toes, checking in with your body and releasing any tension along the way.

Remember to breathe! Move through your neck, front torso, arms, hands, fingers, spinal column, lower back, buttocks, pelvic area, legs, feet, and toes. Directing your mind to release bodily tension releases mental tension as well.

4. Having moved along your entire body in this way, pay close attention. Is there any place that needs additional attention? Return there, and consciously breathe into that area, releasing tension as you exhale. When you feel completely at ease, slowly return your attention to the present.

A variation on this ritual is to tense each part of your body for ten seconds and then let go. You can use this practice anytime, anywhere—serenity now!

PLEASURE-HEALING RITUAL: You Deserve a Break Today

If your circuits are on overload, it's time to pull back and ask yourself why you're so driven. If you don't know whether you're coming or going, it's only a matter of time before some form of intervention takes place to get you to slow down. It might be a failed relationship, an addiction, an accident, or an illness. It's essential that we put ourselves back at the top of our to-do list. Give yourself permission to noodle around a bit. Take back your time. Don't give it all away. In giving ourselves extreme self-care, taking time out to be idle can go a long way toward expelling stress. Disconnect from all the machines and spend the day doing nothing but dancing to your own internal melody, spinning your radio dial, and watching the clouds. Go for a long, meandering walk with no destination in mind. Lie in your backyard hammock and stare at the stars. Watch Swedish adult cinema or Clint Eastwood's spaghetti westerns one after another—whatever floats your boat.

Keep a positive attitude while doing nothing. When you're relaxed, your body is at rest and your mind is open to positive suggestions. If you obsess on a negative thought (especially one that makes you feel guilty for being idle!), ask yourself whether that thought is productive. If the answer is no, tell yourself, "Stop! This is not constructive," and refocus your thinking on a positive affirmation.

You can also visualize. Imagine loading your negative thoughts into a small boat, and then watch the boat drift out to sea and sink. Just remember, when done regularly and with a positive focus, doing nothing reduces stress, improves coping skills, boosts self-confidence and self-worth, and just plain feels good.

PLEASURE-HEALING RITUAL: Hydrotherapy

A delightful ritual and marvelous delivery medium for aromatherapy (which I'll say more about in a later chapter), bathing has long been seen as a ritual synonymous with purifying, cleansing, and calming. Water relaxes tight muscles, rejuvenates sore joints, and stimulates the release of endorphins, leaving one relaxed emotionally and physically. Cultures and spas around the world know this—from the Japanese *onsen* (hot springs) to the clay-laden hot springs in the Ecuadorian Andes to Europe's coastal spas offering heated seawater baths and freshwater mineral ones. Then there's the *hamam* (Turkish bath) found in the Middle East and North Africa. Stateside, spas offer up a delightful selection of hydrotherapies. I've experienced the renowned Kohler Waters Spa in Chicago. With more locations in Kohler, Wisconsin and St. Andrews, Scotland, Kohler's all about water. The "water experiential area" offers a waterfall, whirlpool, several types of showers, and more—heavenly!

See any cleansing ritual as a deep, meditative experience of purification and renewal. Modulate the energy in your environment during this pleasure healing ritual. Light a candle. Awaken and calm the senses through aroma, music, and the like (and, dare I say, a glass of champagne and an organic truffle!). For some of you, it may involve closing your eyes and moving into a deep inner silence. For the adventurous, an energizing shower with alternating hot and cold water will stimulate blood circulation and tone the skin. It's all good!

The pleasure-healing approach allows you to control stress, instead of letting stress control you.

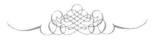

CHAPTER 3

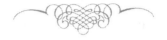

BREATHING LESSONS

Controlling the breath, and thus calming the nerves, is a prerequisite to controlling the mind and the body.

—SWAMI RAMA

Changing your lifestyle to reduce stress is no small task. We're creatures of habit, conditioned bundles of reflexes. This chapter explores a stress-reduction practice universally available to us all: healing breath. Smooth, fluid, natural breathing is an important part of any mindfulness or meditation practice. Breath work is also an important practice in and of itself.

Slow, deep breathing is a profound remedy for stress. If sold by prescription, it'd be the best-selling drug in the world! Some holistic physicians, such as Dr. Andrew Weil, director of the Program in Integrative Medicine and clinical professor of medicine at the

University of Arizona in Tucson, prescribe healing breath as their single-best antistress medicine. In fact, it's my understanding that Dr. Weil considers breathing to be the simplest and most powerful technique for protecting our health and that he has observed that breath control alone lowers blood pressure, stops heart arrhythmias, improves enduring patterns of indigestion, increases overall blood circulation, decreases anxiety, reduces people's need to take addictive antianxiety drugs, and enhances sleep and energy cycles. Smooth, even breathing balances the autonomic nervous system, creating an internal rhythm that nurtures body organs and systems. The *sympathetic* part of the autonomic nervous system is responsible for the fight-or-flight, or stress, response. The *parasympathetic* part of the autonomic nervous system is associated with maintenance and rest. Deep breathing activates this system.

Using breath can instantly tame tension, and you have access to breathing's healing powers at any time. "I *am* breathing," you say. Yes, but what's the quality of your breathing technique, and does it provide the full healing benefits for your mind-body physiology? Learn how to get the most out of every breath.

BREATH IS LIFE

A single wailing breath hails our arrival into the world, just as a single silent one marks our departure from it. In between, we breathe about 23,040 times each day, taking hundreds of millions of breaths over the course of a lifetime. With each inhalation, we take in air molecules that oxygenate our blood and send it coursing through our veins to every bodily cell, simultaneously energizing and relaxing us. And our every exhale makes the grass grow greener, sending carbon dioxide into the environment; releasing metabolic wastes; and detoxifying, purifying, and renewing our mind-body physiology.

At this moment, you're breathing some of the same molecules once breathed by Leonardo da Vinci, Colette, Buddha, William Shakespeare, or whomever else you care to think about. It's amazing that when we release a deep breath, we exhale about ten sextillion air molecules, and it takes about six years for one breath to scatter totally throughout the earth's atmosphere, eventually winding up in such faraway places as Paris, Bombay, or Rio de Janeiro. So my friends, while you may not be able to afford a glamorous stroll along the Champs-Élysées, your breath molecules might do just that.

REMEMBERING HOW TO BREATHE

When you breathe mindfully, your mind, body, and spirit are delightfully intertwined instead of at a standoff. Yet in Western society, few people remember how to breathe correctly. We use only a fraction of our potential respiratory capacity.

Watching a sleeping baby shows us the natural way to breathe. Their abdomens will naturally rise and fall with each breath, making full use of the diaphragm, that broad muscle sandwiched between the lungs and the abdomen. Breathing this way is called diaphragmatic, or "belly," breathing.

As we hold life's stresses within our minds and bodies, we unconsciously keep the diaphragm frozen, resulting in short, shallow breaths. Faced with a constant barrage of stress, our muscles tense and our respiration increases.

Then there's also the old-school rule of "sucking in the gut," a great way to temporarily remove inches from your waistline but a definite detriment to your breathing. Breathing this way makes us shallow chest breathers, causing subtle hyperventilation and great suffering of our bodily systems and mental processes. On the other hand, breathing correctly creates an internal rhythm that keeps all of our mind-body processes functioning in physiological harmony.

Tune In to Your Breath

Check your breathing right now. Put one hand on your chest and one on your abdomen. Inhale and exhale several times. I hope one of your hands moved! You actually want your abdomen to extend outward as you bring in a deep, fluid breath. The abdomen then contracts inward as you exhale. This is what diaphragmatic breathing looks like.

Return to your beginnings and recapture diaphragmatic breathing. Healing breath, or diaphragmatic breathing, is one of the simplest and most powerful ways to decrease the stress response and increase energy in your mind-body physiology. When you draw air down into the lower portion of your lungs, where the oxygen exchange is most efficient, you stop the overflow of the stress hormone cortisol through the bloodstream, and receive efficient delivery of oxygen to the brain, muscles, and organs, optimizing the movement of lymph through the lymph system and enhancing immune-system functioning. Your overall metabolism improves, and with this, digestive, absorptive, and eliminative processes (all gastrointestinal processes) also improve. Your heart rate slows down, blood pressure normalizes, and tense muscles relax, while the busy mind calms down and unhealthy emotional patterns ease up. Deep breathing can also relieve headaches, backaches, stomachaches, and sleeplessness. It helps to normalize the body's release of endorphins, natural painkillers and mood enhancers.

Healing breath also helps addicts kick the habit, whatever the addiction, and may help overcome anxiety and panic disorder. Diaphragmatic breathing may significantly reduce the frequency of hot flashes in menopausal women. Breathing truly is a built-in, organic method for healing whatever ails you. As with all the glorious and balancing mind-body healing practices shared in these pages, we simply need to commit to practicing.

PLEASURE-HEALING RITUAL: Diaphragmatic Breathing

You can do diaphragmatic breathing anytime, anywhere, and it's incredibly simple to master. Just remember to keep it soft, easy, and fluid. For this ritual, give yourself a quiet space where you'll be undisturbed.

Stand, sit up straight, or lie down. For the most efficient flow of the life-force energy, keep your spine aligned. Now let your shoulders melt down away from your ears. Yes, just let go of those trapezius muscles!

Close your eyes if you'd like. Draw in a deep breath through your nose, which is designed to naturally warm and filter every breath. Feel the flow of life-giving energy as it travels into and through the length and depth of your lungs. You'll feel the lower abdomen move outward. Visualize every cell in your body receiving this life-giving energy.

As you naturally exhale (through your nostrils, if possible), your abdomen will move inward. Feel your navel move inward toward the spine. Don't give the exhale short shrift here; exhale fully. (Gulping the next inhale without having fully exhaled contributes to shallow breathing.) A natural part of the relaxation response is directly linked to the out breath. When you fully exhale, your body relaxes more deeply, more deeply calming the mind. Sense the release of all stress you've held in any part of your body, and let this feeling of release wash over you. You'll begin to simultaneously feel a deep sense of relaxation and a heightened flow of energy.

(Note: If you have sinus issues, a deviated septum, or asthma, do the best you can with inhaling and exhaling through your nostrils. If this is difficult, then breathe through your mouth with your lips slightly open. Keep this process soft, not strained.)

Now do ten deep diaphragmatic breaths as outlined. Work toward full breathing with depth, softness, and ease. There shouldn't be any jerking movements. The deeper and easier the breath, the more the torso expands and contracts. With regular practice, this type of breathing can become an everyday habit.

You can heighten the experience by prolonging each inhalation and exhalation or the length of the overall breath-work session. Extending each inhale and exhale to a count of four with a one-second pause between can help create a smooth, fluid, meditative rhythm. Breath work is an integral part of yoga, meditation, and visualization. If you plan to build any of these techniques into your life, be sure to master breathing first.

Moving a step farther along, you can also increase your repertoire of breathing capabilities beyond basic diaphragmatic breathing.

PRANAYAMA: THE SCIENCE OF BREATH

In the eight-limbed path to yoga, *pranayama*, Sanskrit for "the science of breath," is one of the "limbs," or steps. Breath work has been explored and documented for centuries. Pranayama focuses on achieving different results for the mind-body physiology that include calming, cooling, and energizing payoffs. Let's examine a few of them.

PLEASURE-HEALING RITUAL: Nadi Shodhana (Alternate-Nostril Breathing)

Nadi means "channels of circulation," and *shodhana* means "clearing." *Nadi shodhana* helps clear the channels of circulation, which in turn helps center the mind and relieve tension. Although great for anyone, this technique is particularly effective for calming and quieting those who tend to be overactive in mind and body, or anxious and restless when stressed.

Sit in a relaxed, comfortable position with your spine straight. With your mouth closed, use your right-hand ring finger to close off your left nostril. Inhale smoothly and slowly through your right nostril. Release your left nostril while closing off your right nostril with your thumb. Exhale slowly and smoothly out of your left nostril. Now inhale into your left nostril. Breathe diaphragmatically, making the length of each inhalation and exhalation equal. Close off your left nostril and repeat this cycle of exhalation and inhalation into each nostril several times. Try to eventually build up to doing this ritual for several minutes.

PLEASURE-HEALING RITUAL: Sitali Breath (Cooling Breath)

Because this practice is so soothing for the mind-body physiology, it's an excellent choice for pacifying those who tend toward inflammation of any kind, mind or body. If you've just had a disagreement with someone and you're hot under the collar, *sitali* (cooling breath) may help cool you down.

Sit comfortably with your spine straight and eyes closed. Roll your tongue lengthwise to form a tube. The tip of your tongue will protrude slightly from your mouth. Inhale smoothly through your rolled tongue, making a hissing sound. Follow the cool sensation down your throat and into your lungs. (If your tongue won't roll lengthwise, roll its tip back to touch the soft palate. Inhale through closed teeth, making a hissing sound. Continue with the next step.)

Relaxing your tongue and closing your mouth, exhale fully through your nostrils. Generally, the exhale takes slightly longer than the inhale. Repeat five times. Once proficient with this technique, you may want to extend your practice time.

PLEASURE-HEALING RITUAL: Kapalabhati Breath (Breath of Fire)

Translated, *kapalabhati breath* also means "that which makes the head shine." This practice is invigorating, so it's a great choice anytime you feel lethargic, fatigued, or depressed. It's very effective for balancing the "earth" energy (when you're too grounded to the earth and need to be stimulated, or energized; in an unbalanced state, "heaviness" predominates so that one is stagnant, or complacent, as in the "couch potato"), because it tends to stimulate the abdominal muscles and digestive organs, massage the internal organs and spinal column, and increase circulation of bodily fluids.

Sit comfortably with your spine straight and eyes closed. Place the palms of both hands on your abdomen. Inhale slowly and passively. Now vigorously and forcefully exhale through your nose while drawing your stomach tightly inward. Repeat this passive inhalation and forceful exhalation ten times. Once comfortable with this technique, you can use it for up to one minute. (Don't use kapalabhati breath if you're pregnant or have untreated heart disease.)

PLEASURE-HEALING RITUAL: Ujjayi Breath (Victorious Breath)

In Sanskrit, *ujjayi* means "control arising from the process of expansion." Ujjayi breath enhances the ventilation of the lungs, removes congestion, calms the nerves, and energizes the entire body. This practice helps vitalize the whole body. In my clinical yoga practice, I've used this technique with great success for a variety of chronic issues, including asthma and fibromyalgia. Because it creates an obvious sound, it's an ideal technique to use when performing yoga, since this sound gently reminds you to keep breathing while holding or moving through postures.

In ujjayi the sound made while inhaling and exhaling is "ha." To get the hang of this, first try breathing in and out with your mouth open. With the glottis (the opening between the vocal cords in the larynx) at the back of your throat constricted, inhale while making the "ha" sound. Then exhale, making the "ha" sound. If you sound like Darth Vader, you're doing it right! Whether done for ten breaths, ten minutes, or throughout a half-hour yoga practice, ujjayi is a surefire way to conjure free-flowing energy with full awareness.

PLEASURE-HEALING RITUAL: Two-to-One Breathing

Two-to-one breathing is one of the most profoundly calming techniques, especially effective if sound slumber eludes you, but it can also be used whenever you feel exceptionally stressed out. It stimulates the parasympathetic nervous system, which slows down the heartbeat, lowers the blood pressure, and creates harmonious brain-wave patterns.

Consciously slow your exhalation down to twice as long as your inhalation. For instance, try counting to three on the inhale and to six on the exhale. Contract your abdominal muscles (especially the transversus abdominis muscle, just above the pubic bone) to help increase the exhalation. Try to make each breath as smooth and even as possible, without any pauses or shakiness.

If you're having trouble going to sleep, lie on your back and do eight two-to-one breaths, then turn on your right side and do sixteen breaths, and finally turn on your left side and do thirty-two breaths. Chances are that you won't finish this experience before drifting off to la-la land.

Deep, gentle breathing is one of the most effortless highs you'll ever experience. Try it right now, and often. There are few things in life as pleasurable as this gentle dive into tranquility.

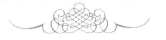

CHAPTER 4

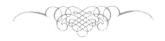

JUST SAY "OM"

The quieter you become, the more you can hear.

—RAM DASS

Many healers call meditation the ultimate and most important practice for realizing optimal well-being, that is, our wholeness. Quite frankly, you can try any other practice, treatment, or therapy, but unless you experience the awakening to your true self born of regular meditation practice, the transformation and deep healing that move us toward wholeness may go unrealized or be stunted.

WHY MEDITATE?

To successfully establish a practice, which can be challenging, you have to *want* to meditate. My greatest wish right now is that this chapter serve as the springboard for you to dive in. A meditation practice is nonnegotiable; you just have to do it. Long an integral part of all the world's great wisdom traditions, meditation conveys great richness, depth, and mysticism. Whether in the Vedic or Yogic tradition, or in Buddhism, Sufism, Judaism, or Christianity, it's universally affirmed that this form of spiritual practice is essential to spiritual awakening.

In our time-starved, need-for-speed society where we tend to ignore internal signals and let external ones rule, it's essential to give ourselves time to break free and listen to spirit. Meditation practice can bring us to this place. It frees us from the bondage of our egocentricities and the external influences that prevent us from connecting with the soul, that pure-consciousness layer of our being where infinite possibilities reside.

BECOME WHO YOU TRULY ARE

The pure-consciousness layer of our being is where we access our true source of balance, fulfillment, and well-being. Meditation allows us to experience this layer consistently so that profound shifts begin to take place in our lives. We begin to understand who we really are, why we're here, and how we can serve with heightened creativity, intuition, compassion, vitality, energy, and bliss. A daily commitment to this practice infuses our mind-body physiology with stability, flexibility, and great resiliency. Considered by many healers to be the *it* skill of the twenty-first century, resiliency is our ability to get over, through, and beyond the challenges we face and come out on the other side unscathed and stronger for it.

Meditation practitioners attest to the many benefits meditation offers: peace of mind, release of bodily tension, deeper concentration, mental clarity, increased energy and vitality, heightened optimism, and the ability to remain calm in all situations. Meditation is also a prime pump for compassion, and tremendously enhances our ability to express greater empathy, understanding, forgiveness, nonjudgment, and loving-kindness. In Eastern wisdom traditions, meditation has long been a way of achieving bliss, fostering self-actualization, and exploring higher levels of consciousness.

Commit to a meditation practice with a personal statement of intent: "I intend to commune with spirit today and every day." Say it out loud with relish and conviction. Sing it, if you'd like. Show yourself how serious you are about your commitment.

SILENCE **IS** GOLDEN

In meditation we experience one of life's great favors: silence. When we can carve out bits of time throughout our day to intentionally be in silence, we become more present in each moment as we live our lives. We begin to mindfully make more life-affirming choices and thus sow the seeds that allow us to live a balanced life. We heighten our ability to communicate with others, express ideas creatively, become more compassionate and tolerant, unconditionally love ourselves and others, and strive for the higher meaning in life. *Meditation is a sacred gift we give to ourselves.*

MEDITATION: THE ULTIMATE HEALTH CARE

Among its numerous health benefits, meditation creates greater brain-wave coherence, allowing the brain to communicate better with the rest of the body. During meditation the brain and the body calm down enough to work together. Constancy and synchronicity among brain-wave patterns bring greater clarity of thought, enhanced intuition, creativity, and memory recall. Along with quieting down the overactive mind, meditation may lower blood pressure, slow down the heartbeat, and calm the central nervous system. By virtue of all this, it may provide a powerful boost to the immune system. Meditation has also been used to treat high cholesterol, high blood pressure, and headaches.

Meditators have a thicker cerebral cortex than non-meditators. More brain matter means higher levels of mental acuity and activity. Meditation can rewire brain circuitry, knitting together dissimilar brain circuits to make us more stress resilient. And on the happiness front, meditation significantly shifts brain waves from right-prefrontal cortex to left-prefrontal cortex, where positive emotions and optimism reside.

Meditation may also regulate hormones and increase levels of serotonin, the brain's feel-good neurotransmitter. Integrative physicians recommend meditation for its mental-health benefits, such as relief from anxiety and depression (by lowering levels of cortisol), increased resistance to potential emotional disturbances, relief from compulsive behaviors and addictions, and better rest and sleep.

MEDITATION AND THE RELAXATION RESPONSE

Meditation can elicit the *relaxation response*, a term coined by Dr. Herbert Benson, one of the most renowned researchers on meditation and Mind/Body Medical Institute associate, professor of medicine at Harvard Medical School, director emeritus of the Benson-Henry institute for Mind/Body Medicine at Massachusetts General Hospital in Boston, and author of the best-selling classic *The Relaxation Response*. Meditation slows down the heart rate, respiration, and brain waves so that brain-wave electrical activity becomes more coherent, muscles relax, and the effects of stress hormones diminish. Meditation allows you to fluidly take your awareness into a deep inner silence. When this happens, mental activity decreases along with overall biochemical activity, giving the body a profound rest deeper than sleep. As we train the disturbed and distracted mind to become more focused, we gain tremendous power. With the resulting heightened awareness and mental clarity, we're able to concentrate better and thus do just about anything more effectively.

THE MEDITATION MENU

Meditation comes in a variety of "flavors": concentrative, passive, mindfulness, loving-kindness, visualization, and movement, to name but a few. I teach two major practices in this chapter: concentrative meditation and loving-kindness meditation.

At its heart, meditation refers to time spent in quiet introspection, and however you can best accomplish this will become your form of meditation. You may go for long walks, do yoga or tai chi, pray, or use a mantra (a concentrative technique where you direct your mind with single-pointed focus to an object of your attention). You can write in a journal, pore over devotional books or scriptural verse, or listen to some form of inspirational music, letting your imagination and feelings carry you more deeply into it. As long as a given activity takes you to a place of calm, heightened awareness and energy, clarity of mind, and joyfulness and positivity, then you're meditating.

Concentrative Meditation

In essence, meditation (in its purest, most traditional form) is the process of focusing your awareness. This level of concentration is significant in how it trains the mind and elicits the relaxation response. Concentrative meditation is giving your single-pointed focus to the object of your attention, for example, repeating a mantra (Sanskrit for "instrument of the mind") such as *om* or other sounds often translated to mean "peace," such as *shalom*, *amen*, or *salaam*. A mantra could also be a word or sound of your choosing, or simple observation of the breath.

The healing breath we discussed earlier is a natural segue into meditation, because the simplest of meditative techniques is concentration on the breath. Why, your concentration may even rest in your awareness of Self or your thoughts, in a mindfulness meditation. You may also choose to chant; closely watch a candle's flame; use a rosary or mala beads; gaze at sacred visual symbols such as a statue, picture, mandala (a design used in Hinduism and Buddhism containing concentric geometric forms, images of deities, and so on, symbolizing the universe, totality, or wholeness), or yantra (geometric design whose complex numeric construction includes geometric shapes, colors, and symbols, each part of which has specific and significant meaning right down to a single dot); meditate on a color or a gem's energetic patterns; and so on.

Using a Mantra

A mantra is looked upon as an instrument of the mind (*man* means "mind," and *tra* means "instrument"). In our sound-bite culture, one might use "mantra" as shorthand for a mission statement ("get it done," "seize the day," or "open and release"), however trivial ("I *must* find shoes to match this dress"). In the Yogic tradition in which the term originated, a *mantra* is a Sanskrit syllable, word, or verse that, when repeated, creates sonic vibrations that bring us to the deepest, most-silent realm of our being, encouraging spiritual awakening. You can choose your own mantra or be assigned one, as in Transcendental Meditation and Primordial Sound Meditation instruction (the Chopra Center for Well-Being's approach). If you choose your own mantra, pick a word that means something to you and is soothing. It can be your child's name, or the word "one," "peace," or "love." Enjoyment of the word's sound and connection to its meaning contribute to a mantra's power.

PLEASURE-HEALING RITUAL: Concentrative Meditation

Try to give yourself the gift of meditation every single day. Personally, I enjoy meditating for twenty minutes at dawn and dusk, the times when our circadian rhythms (the twenty-four-hour daily cycle) are most calm and peaceful. But consistency is more important than duration. Begin with a few minutes and build to longer sessions as you experience the tremendous benefits.

Choose a quiet and comfortable place. Creating a tranquil atmosphere softens the mind so you can more readily focus. If your meditation space is in your own personal setting, make it special with comfortable cushions to support your body as needed. Since this is a sacred atmosphere where you'll go to connect with spirit, enhance it with a candle, incense, or nature or ambient sounds on CDs (for example, drumming, chanting, toning, and so on). In your workplace, do the best you can to find your "space." But also trust that as you become a long-term meditator, you'll become quite adept at meditating anytime and anywhere.

To calm and center yourself before beginning meditation, consider doing a few minutes of diaphragmatic breathing, alone or with a few yoga postures, to begin quieting the overactive mind. Make yourself feel comfortable, preferably with your spinal column aligned, whether lying down, or seated on the floor or in a chair. (Our spinal cord houses the central nervous system and, when healthy and unrestricted, is a column of flowing biological energy.) Close your eyes so that your brain can more readily stop process-ing information coming from the senses. Concentrate, breathing smoothly and naturally. Don't try to modulate or control your breath in any way.

Begin saying your mantra or chosen word to yourself with every out breath. (If you're working with a phrase or verse, you can use the entire breath.) This rhythm will help you to focus. Repeat your mantra again and again. This will require your concentration. If thoughts come into your mind, gently and nonjudgmentally watch them come and go, and bring your attention back to the repetition of your word. Do this for as long as time permits, remembering that even a few moments can benefit, with longer meditation sessions reaping the most significant and deep benefits over time. Gently, open your eyes and bring your awareness back to your surroundings.

Alternatively, you can also choose to simply become aware of your breath, so that breathing, in itself, becomes the object of your concentration. Become aware of your breathing. Breathe deeply, smoothly, and naturally, paying attention to the feel of your breath as you inhale and exhale. Feel the sensations. Inhale through your nostrils to warm and purify the air as it comes into your lungs. Exhale through your nostrils or mouth. Continue to witness the inflow and outflow of your breath. Your belly moves out on the inhale and contracts inward on the exhale. Don't try to modulate or control your breath in any way. It's okay to get distracted by thoughts floating through your mind, sounds in the surrounding environment, or sensations in the body. Let them come and go like migrating birds or clouds drifting through the sky, and bring your attention back to your breath. Be innocent and gentle with yourself through this process, and don't force it in any way. Continue this process for up to twenty minutes or even beyond; whatever your pleasure—healing pleasure, that is!

Am I Doing This Right?

I've just outlined one of the most traditional ways to meditate. Please understand that you can meditate wherever you are, at any time, and in any way you choose. No matter where, when, why, or how you meditate, know that there's no wrong way to do it. If you find yourself falling asleep, it's okay. It indicates that you're tired! If you find yourself fending off a barrage of thoughts, it's okay. It indicates that you have a lot on your mind and probably need to release these thoughts before they turn into harmful stress. Let the thoughts come and go. Be their "witness"; don't judge them or let them influence you to act on them in any way. Acknowledge them, but stay calmly detached from them. You can talk to yourself about this: "What an interesting thought. I'll think about you later. Good-bye for now." Then return to the object of your attention: your mantra, word, or breath.

Be consistent, and remember that ongoing practice brings the most profound benefits, because the mind is wily and resists settling down at first. As for finding the right way to access the silence we discussed, trust me, you'll find it. All you need to do is show up with the intention, and you'll experience an awakening to the miracle of existence. Over time your life will become a continual meditation, 24 hours a day, 7 days a week, 365 days a year. And yes, this *is* possible!

Loving-Kindness Meditation

I saw a bumper sticker not too long ago that said, "Love is our soul purpose." In this spirit, I offer you the practice of loving-kindness meditation. Loving-kindness meditation has been taught through the ages as a balm for the soul, opening the heart and conjuring deep feelings of compassion, peace, and acceptance, as well as the healing force of unconditional love, first toward ourselves and then to all life. Though loving-kindness meditation comes from the Buddhist tradition, anyone can appreciate it. I've particularly been influenced by the Insight Meditation Society and one of its founders, Sharon Salzberg.

In a hurting world, loving-kindness meditation can open us up to the infinite possibilities for eliciting deep heartfelt love and soothing difficult emotions. *Make no mistake: love is the most powerful force there is and, when practiced with full intention, it can help overcome any suffering we may experience.* Buddha taught that the mind is naturally radiant and pure. It's when the dark and turbulent forces invade the mind that we suffer. Anger, violence, greed, disgust, guilt, and resentment are all different forms of pain. Cultivating a deep sense of love and understanding—first toward ourselves, then toward all living beings, and finally to all of creation—can transform our experience of pain. We become an open, accepting, and expansive vessel of light and love toward life's pleasures and pain. From this place of wholeness and love, we can quell our fear and learn to embrace all that is. Having a loving mind provides great freedom to shift with the tides, to be resilient, so you can observe joy one moment and grief the next, without becoming overwhelmed by the change.

Buddha said, "You can search throughout the entire universe for someone who is more deserving of your love and affection than you are yourself, and that person is not to be found anywhere. You yourself, as much as anybody in the entire universe, deserve your love and affection." At our core, we're pure goodness and love personified—and we can nurture this into full-blown existence. Seeing this goodness doesn't mean we should ignore difficult aspects. Rather, our purpose is to create an energetic shift through an intention to focus on the positive. As we focus, we forge wholeness within ourselves and true interconnectedness with others.

Pleasure-Healing Ritual: Loving-Kindness Meditation

Sit or lie down in a comfortable position, with an aligned, or neutral, spine. Gently close your eyes. Bring your attention to your heart chakra area (one of seven energetic centers along the spine from tailbone to crown), emanating from the center of the chest. Breathe in and out through your heart center, as if all mind-body experience happens from there. Witness the inflow and outflow of the breath. The heart, mind, and body will begin to soften, relaxing and releasing any held stress. With full presence, witness yourself in this moment.

Begin with loving-kindness toward yourself. If you sense any blockages or negative feelings, imagine dropping beneath them to the place where your only desire is to nurture yourself, and be safe and well. You can use the phrases shared here or your own. See if any positive statements bubble up from your heart center that express deep desires for yourself yet are expansive enough to include all of creation.

Here are some possible phrases: *"May I be safe and protected from harm. May I be deeply joyful. May I be peacefully at ease. May I be healthy and strong."* While saying these phrases, consider Buddha's guidance to see yourself as a beloved child, evoking tremendous care, warmth, and tenderness.

Gently repeat the phrases again and again, letting the feelings that arise permeate the layers of your being. Do this for one minute, five minutes, or twenty minutes, whatever your time allows. If your mind wanders off, don't worry. Nonjudgmentally and gently witness your lapsed attention in this moment, and bring it back to focus on the phrases. You can even abbreviate these phrases; for example, *"May I be safe, deeply joyful, peacefully at ease, healthy, and strong."* Be in the moment with these positive statements, feeling them resonate through your mind and body. Feel the love!

Now think of someone in your life whom you care deeply about, perhaps someone who's cared for you or inspired you. This could be a parent, dear friend, or teacher. Visualize this person and feel his or her presence. Now direct loving-kindness to this person: *"May you be safe, deeply joyful, peacefully at ease, healthy, and strong."* Repeat the phrase again and again as time permits. Really tune in to the broadcasting of these feelings.

Next, consider someone who's having a difficult time in his or her life right now, whatever the situation. Imagine being with this person. Feel his or her presence. Now offer loving-kindness to this person: "May you *be safe, deeply joyful, peacefully at ease, healthy, and strong.*"

The next step opens the heart beyond the scope of those we generally share our love with. Think of someone in your life who plays a more neutral role, whether a cashier at the grocery store, a bus driver, a dry-cleaner attendant, or a gas-station clerk. Imagine being with this person, and feel his or her presence. Now offer loving-kindness to this person.

We've come this far. Now we're ready to expand our loving-kindness outward to all of creation. Send out your boundless love without reservation: "May all *living beings be safe, deeply joyful, peacefully at ease, healthy, and strong.*" This unbounded, loving energy will deeply heal and transform you and all of creation. Vary the phrases or people to whom you send your loving-kindness as circumstances require.

Gently come out of this meditation, taking this energy with you as you embark on your daily activities. Use this practice anywhere: on trains, planes, and automobiles; or at the doctor's office, a business meeting, or home. As you practice it among others, you'll immediately feel a wonderful connection to them. Deep love and affection will grow unbounded, along with the healing benefits!

MEDITATION: AT THE HEART OF TRUE HEALING

Along with my daily breathing practices, meditation is how I stay in the moment, reduce stress, find inner peace, and remain the optimist, even in the face of tremendous challenge. You have to really want these benefits in your life before you can make a true commitment to meditation. If you do commit, I promise you that meditation will rock your world. The awakening to "what is" is quite powerful and awe inspiring. It will change everything about how you experience every facet of your life. Again and again, you'll want to recapture the glimpse of your soul that you experience during meditation. It becomes your new reality. Meditation brings on a spiritual awareness that sweeps over us, leaving us trembling before the presence of a mystery almost too vivid and beautiful to bear. Once you've experienced this, there's really no turning back. Just as with physical exercise, you'll find that you don't want to compromise your meditation time. It will become as important and integral to your day as bathing, eating, physical activity, and sleeping.

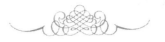

CHAPTER 5

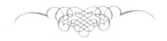

Nourishing Wisdom

Tell me what you eat, and I will tell you what you are.

—Anthelme Brillat Savarin

Bill Cosby wrote a book titled *I Am What I Ate . . . and I'm Frightened!!!* Well, we certainly shouldn't be frightened; however, we *do* become the food we eat. The quality and quantity, as well as surrounding aura, of last night's dinner mixed with our DNA become the constellation of molecules, cells, tissues, and organs that makes up our bodies, minds, and moods. The result can be a symphonic masterpiece or discordant junk. Personally, I'll go for the symphonic goodness any day. How about you? So let's explore approaches that help you get there, approaches infused with a spa sensibility.

Eating brings pleasure to our palates and satisfaction to our souls. The spa world understands this premise. The principles of spa cuisine can offer extraordinary guidance. Some spas even offer cooking classes with one of the spa's chefs and, in many cases, a nutritionist. Naturally, in these settings mindfulness, high-level nutrition, exquisite freshness, taste, and presentation, as well as portion control come into play. As in all life-affirming practices, the beginning emphasis is on fostering a deeper mindfulness toward the sacred act of eating and the sensual nature of taking nourishment, rather than the "right" caloric intake, ratios of carbs to fats to proteins, lists of "approved" foods and recipes, and the like. Truly, the answer to healthful and fully delightful eating is inside every one of us. We just need to slow down and pay attention to the *nourishing wisdom* in each and every one of us.

WHY WE EAT

We experience some of life's greatest pleasures through our sense of taste. Yes, we eat food for nourishment, but eating also brings us a veritable buffet of additional pleasures.

Nourishing the Body

Healthful food choices advance the flow of the life-force energy through your body, raising your vibration and healing capacity. Eating a balanced diet of nutritious, delicious organic and whole foods gives you tremendous energy; a strong, resilient body; and greater immunity to emotional and physical toxins. Thoughtful, high-level nutrition can prevent inflammation, a major cause of degenerative disease and aging. By selecting foods that fortify your arteries and veins, you're better able to absorb and use nutrients. Every cell in your body works in physiological harmony, doing the right job, clearing the way for astonishing well-being, not to mention glowing skin; shiny, lustrous hair; strong nails; and radiant eyes (how's this for a dynamic daily positive affirmation and creative visualization?).

Connecting with Others

For many of us, meals also provide a nurturing and blissful way to connect with others. What would the TV series *Seinfeld* have been without Jerry, Elaine, George, and Kramer kibitzing over their meal at the local coffee shop? Or how about the camaraderie found over a brew at *Cheers*? "Breaking bread" with others *is* a ritual and an honor. Be grateful for this soulful connection. Infuse it with your thoughtful presence; don't let it be a haphazard occurrence. Whether it's two friends sharing lunch, an entire village feasting in celebration, extended families reuniting, or business associates sealing a deal over breakfast, every one of us can create our own version of this feel-good ritual.

If you're dining solo, make the experience a sensual one: light a candle, arrange flowers, play beautiful music, have framed photos of loved ones close at hand, and serve yourself a delicious meal on a beautiful plate. Perhaps set another place setting for a distant loved one, or feed your pet, if you have one, at the same time you take your meal. Express gratitude and then eat every delectable morsel of your meal with full awareness.

Nourishing the Spirit

Food also represents an expression of our spirituality; for example, the bread and wine of Christian communion; the unleavened bread and herbs at Jewish Passover; the harvest offerings in Native American ceremonies; and the bountiful spreads at life-altering events, such as births, weddings, and deaths. Even during life's more private moments, food can nourish the soul. A simple snack or meal can intensify romantic interludes, encourage fabulous connection, fuel flirtatious energy, bring into focus great fortune in life, and ultimately provide a host of additional potentially sensual or enlightening experiences.

PLEASURE-HEALING RITUAL: Nourishing Intention

Think about the last time that eating food was a sacred ritual of engaging with others. Reflect on this for a moment. Make it your goal to bring this sacredness into all your eating experiences. And, yes, this begins with a powerful statement of intention: "As I eat, I'm present and thankful for how my food choices nourish me." Come up with your own intention each day. Make it present tense, and remember, don't be wishy-washy! We program our nervous system with our thoughts and words.

Emotional Hunger

Eating mindfully is one of the most powerful ways to nurture our bodies and souls, but too often we allow our hectic lifestyles to twist and deform this most basic human act. Indeed, food may become a metaphor. Today, many overindulge in unhealthy types or quantities of food, desperately hoping to feed a deep spiritual hunger. Though this explanation is oversimplified, anorexia, an act of self-starvation, is often triggered by the need to gain control over one's life, while obesity can result when one forgets to feed the heart with love and attempts to fill the resulting void with junk-food binges. Whether famished for things or experiences, starving souls will always seek to fill up somehow.

Many exhilarating and soulful experiences in life can feed us: spirituality, relationships, vocation (or more succinctly, right livelihood) physical activities, and leisure pursuits. When we're satisfied in these areas of life, food takes its rightful place as a source of nutrition and energy at life's banquet.

Have you ever been in the most passionate stage of love? It's so exhilarating, wouldn't you say? The senses are as vibrantly alive as can be. The magic of intimacy in a lover's touch and the feelings of excitement sustain us. Gazing into your lover's eyes feels as if you're floating on air. Or remember being a child and playing outside for hours. Maybe your mom called you to come in for dinner, but you weren't hungry at all. The exuberance of play had all your attention. It was your "food" for that window of time. Such moments and feelings demonstrate that *everything* can be nutrition. There are thousands of life experiences that "feed" us physically, mentally, emotionally, and spiritually.

Love, touch, intimacy, play, creativity, self-expression, achievement, adventure, and spirituality are all essential forms of nourishment. Keep them in balance with the actual food hunger you feel. Reflect on what "feeds" your soul, and intend to integrate these experiences into your life as best you can. The extent to which you consciously do this determines how pleasurable and balanced your life feels.

INTUITIVE EATING

Each of us holds an innate, intuitive intelligence so powerful that it can tell us how to heal and prevent illness. In opening up to spirit, we open up to our intuition, a vital part of our wisdom. As we learn to trust this inner sense and its messages, stress and anxiety lessen, emotional blocks clear, and healing processes accelerate. As we eat intuitively, we become exquisitely tuned in to what our mind-body physiology feels, needs, and desires; this is our nourishing wisdom.

Chew on This

Bring these aspects of nutrition into your consciousness: nourishment to fuel and fortify mind and body, human connection, spirituality, and misplaced dependence on food to feed the soul. As you do this, remember that knowledge is power. Learn how food affects you. Listen to your inner yearnings. "Do I want the tuna fish or the chicken-salad sandwich? The fresh fruit salad or that dense piece of chocolate cheesecake?" This becomes a regular dialogue with yourself, and eventually, you become very good at weeding out unhealthy choices. Pay attention to how food makes you feel, because it will fiercely affect your energy and moods. As you learn to eat with love and awareness, visualize how food nourishes both your mind and body. If you let this be your focus every time you take a bite, whether it's a tiny snack or a great feast, your life will be transformed.

The Intuitive vs. the Stress Eater

Become an intuitive eater. Mindfully eat delicious high-quality food—but slowly, in moderation, and with great pleasure. Intuitive eating is paying attention to the cues your body sends you, listening to its signals. Learn to feel hunger, and feed yourself the most flavorful, healthy food on the planet rather than react to stress, going for the latest dietary advice or bouncing from fad to fad. A yo-yo, on-again off-again diet mentality is counterproductive and, for many, a failure.

Don't get caught up in the diet mentality. The deprivation we feel creates even more stress, which causes more of the stress hormone cortisol to circulate through our blood, depositing fat in the belly area, among other places. If chronically stressed, your body keeps churning out cortisol, causing you to continually reach for sugary, starchy, and fat-laden foods. And with this, blood-sugar levels rise dramatically, then come crashing down, with the resulting fatigue. Insulin is released into the bloodstream to handle the blood sugar, over time creating insulin resistance, a precursor to diabetes. If the energy from this food intake is *not* spent on an activity, the fat deposits itself in the belly area. It's a vicious cycle but one we can control as we learn techniques for managing stress, including healthful eating. This will also resensitize your taste buds to become more tuned in to the natural and satisfying flavors of nutrient-dense, real foods. You become an intuitive eater rather than a stress eater.

Opt for whole, unprocessed foods. They should also be rich in protein, complex carbohydrates, healthy fats, and vitamins and minerals. Make whole grains, beans, nuts, and fresh vegetables the mainstay of your diet. They contain fiber and nutrients that keep blood-sugar levels stable, and they make neurotransmitters in the brain that help you feel good. And with this, you'll lose your appetite for cheap, calorie-dense, sugary, and starchy processed food.

Balance proteins, fats, and complex carbs with every meal or snack. High refined-carb diets rapidly raise and then lower blood sugar, wreaking havoc with insulin levels. Protein and healthy fats in the diet help slow down carb absorption, keeping blood-sugar levels steady. If we don't get enough protein, fat, and fiber, our bodies crank out even more cortisol, triggering cravings and the added burden of guilt.

Don't skip meals. You'll be ravenous, and reach for sugary and high-carb foods. Eat smaller, more-frequent meals that emphasize fresh, whole foods. Grazing throughout the day, at three-hour intervals (five small meals over the course of the day), may be the best way to keep the metabolism humming along optimally.

And please, break your fast! Eat a protein-rich breakfast, such as eggs or nut butter on whole-grain toast or with fresh fruit. Skipping breakfast or eating a bagel on the run wreaks havoc with your blood sugar, making you more sensitive to stress. If you drink coffee first thing in the morning, your adrenal glands release cortisol into your bloodstream, jacking you up without any high-quality food to stabilize or buffer the caffeine's effect on your system.

Physical activity plays into this equation. It not only brightens the mood but also reduces cortisol and improves overall stress resilience. And weight training not only provides cortisol control but also revs up our metabolism, helping us to tone up and slim down at the same time.

Get a handle on the stress. Create pockets of peace throughout your day. Sidestep stress whenever you can, and avoid situations that push your buttons.

And last but not least, supplement wisely with antistress nutrients:

- Magnesium and the B vitamins are well known for their relaxation and mood-lifting benefits. Take 400 mg of magnesium and at least 100 percent of the recommended daily allowance of the B vitamins every day.

- The herb holy basil reduces cortisol and helps our bodies adapt to stress. Experts recommend 400 mg two times a day. Also called *tulsi*, it comes in tea form as well as capsules.

- If a stressful event is on the horizon or you've just experienced a traumatic event, try L-theanine. It's an amino acid in green tea that controls cortisol and helps you relax within thirty minutes without any side effects. It also increases GABA—a neurotransmitter in the brain that helps you stay calm and focused. You can take 50 to 150 mg.

Consult with your physician if you want to add supplements to your daily diet, especially if you're on any type of prescription medicines.

Tune In to Your Eating Habits

Think about your eating habits. Reflect on and see them for what they really are. Consider a typical day at home, work, and play. From awareness, change and transformation can happen. The next time you take a lunch break, visit your favorite restaurant, or prepare a meal at home, ask yourself, "Will these food choices make me feel good? Will they optimize my energy levels and, ultimately, my health and well-being?" Eventually, with your knowledge of the fundamentals of healthy eating and your desire for tasty, whole foods, you'll reply to your own questions with a resounding yes!

PLEASURE-HEALING RITUAL: Assess Your Diet

Write your answers to the following questions in your journal. Take note of the circumstances or the "why" surrounding your answers.

- Generally, how many meals do you eat per day?

- How many of these meals are eaten outside your home?

- Do you snack a great deal?

- What sort of snacks do you eat?

- Do you try to have protein, complex carbohydrates, and healthy fats at every meal or snack?

- Do you carefully plan and prepare your meals, whether taken at home or to work?

- Do you cook meals from scratch? How does this make you feel?

- Do you buy precooked meals?

- Do you understand boxed, canned, and bagged food labels?

- Do you purchase certified-organic foods?

- How often do you add sugar, salt, or butter to your food?

- How often do you use fresh herbs and spices?

- Does your typical daily menu need a little TLC?

Jot down a few ways to achieve better eating habits that will work for you.

PLEASURE-HEALING RITUAL: Take Inventory

Make a grocery-shopping list that supports your intention to eat as deliciously and healthfully as possible: organic olive oil, whole-grain bread and pasta, brown rice, raw nut butters, a variety of multicolored veggies for salads, fresh or frozen organic berries, low-fat yogurt, wild-caught Alaskan or smoked salmon, natural or organic chicken, and so on.

PLEASURE-HEALING RITUAL: Reinvent the Meal

Write down all the foods you ate at your last meal. If you used any boxed, canned, or bagged foods, write down the ingredients printed on the container label (note any chemicals in the food). No one's testing you, so be honest! Underline the foods that don't serve you well. Now describe a similar meal or snack, replacing the energy-depleting or downright unhealthy items with good alternatives. For example, if you had nachos with fake cheese, try replacing this meal with homemade quesadillas and salsa—all organic, of course.

PLEASURABLE EATING

It's important to understand that healthy eating is not about deprivation but, rather, about appreciating and eating high-quality food. You can have that decadent dessert, a steak from grass-fed beef, a glass of fine wine, a plate of pasta, and some freshly baked bread. Mindfully enjoy these delectable treats, but make sure that they're whole, organic choices wherever possible and that they're part of an overall balanced diet and lifestyle. Also strive to purchase locally or regionally grown foods, visit your local farmers market, and certainly get to know your local farmers. Why, you could even grow your own food, whether in a plot out back or a pot on your windowsill. Doing so creates a vital and sacred connection with our food. It's the mindless overconsumption of foods we have no connection to—foods that are chemically grown and heavily processed, and void of the life-force energy—that bring our greatest problems.

The Flavor of Life: True Exploration

While we're on the subject of enjoying the natural, unadulterated deliciousness of our foods, let's also discuss stretching our palate a bit. We need to eat as wide a variety of foods as possible to optimize our nutrition. This sounds reasonable enough, but how about broadening your definition of variety by eating foods you've never tried before? Did you know that the world provides over 50,000 edible plants but we eat only about 150 of them as part of our standard diet? Twenty of these account for about 90 percent of our food. Three of them—rice, corn, and wheat—make up half of our diet. By variety, I mean really push your horizons. Have you ever been to an Indian, Thai, Ethiopian, Greek, or Moroccan restaurant? Have you ever ordered the rice taffel at an Indonesian restaurant or sat at a Japanese sushi bar and ordered from the sushi chef? These cultures really know how to eat a diverse selection of foods, and the sauces, garnishes, and side bowls are simply amazing!

Having had the opportunity to travel to the farthest corners of the globe, I've tasted (though sometimes just a bite) some of the most unusual foods, from fried grasshoppers to monkey brain to whale blubber. Every culture has its own distinct idea of what constitutes an enjoyable, nutritious diet.

Variety Is the Spice of Life

You can also experiment with familiar foods prepared in new and different ways. Here's a personal example: I enjoy juicing my breakfast in the morning, at least one to two pounds of organic veggies and sometimes a small amount of fruit added in for extra sweetness. I add a bit of essential fatty acids (the good fats) in flaxseed oil and, sometimes, unsweetened coconut for extra flavor, and change the veggie and fruit selections as desired. Juicing allows you to assimilate the maximum amount of nutrients from your veggies and fruit, so drinking this morning nectar provides a vitamin-packed way to start the day as well as an amazing energy high—pure brain food, this! I'm also big on smoothies for breakfast. Low-fat dairy, soy, rice, or oat milk with frozen or fresh fruits, flaxseed oil, a serving of whey powder, and wow!—what a nutrient-packed way to start the day, keeping your blood sugar, thus energy levels, steady throughout your morning. You can create your own recipes, including fruit juice if desired or adding "green" foods, such as spirulina, wheatgrass, or chlorella (huge detoxifiers and immune boosters). I much prefer blending these concoctions at home, because I can control the ingredients and it's more economical. If you do choose to go to the local smoothie or juice bar, use caution, because many of their ingredients include simple sugars, high-fructose corn syrup (so pervasive in our foods and *so* bad for us), and various non-organic ingredients. If you'd like to learn more about juicing or creating your own smoothies, there are many wonderful books and websites to get you started.

PLEASURE-HEALING RITUAL: Welcome New Culinary Delights

On your next trip to the grocers, resolve to bring one or two new tastes home with you that you've never tried before. If you're a meat eater, go beyond the usual, and try nutritious organ meats, such as tongue, liver, kidney, or giblets. Or try unusual meats, such as ostrich, venison, buffalo, or goat. Buy all-natural and organic whenever possible.

Perhaps you've experimented with the greens of kale, mustard, beet, endive, escarole, or chard. Try a variety of unusual veggies, such as kohlrabi, artichoke, sunchoke, yam, or Chinese cabbage. Dabble in root vegetables, such as turnip or parsnip. Try different grains, perhaps quinoa, amaranth, barley, spelt, or kamut. Try wild or basmati rice. Enjoy tahini (sesame butter), and almond or hemp butters as an alternative to peanut butter. Add new herbs and spices to your pantry: lemongrass, cardamom, turmeric, ginseng, cilantro, saffron, sage, or curry. Buy exotic fruits, such as kiwi, mango, papaya, star, or tangelo. Look for new cheeses such as goat (Buche de Chevre is heavenly!), Asiago, serat (made in Afghanistan from sheep's milk), Gruyère, or Camembert. Try edible flowers, such as nasturtium for its peppery flavor and surprisingly sweet carnation petals or sorrel flowers for a tart, lemony taste. This is pleasure, pleasure, and more pleasure!

Gaining ground in gourmet and spa circles is the concept of *terroir* (pronounced tare-WAHR), a French term that loosely translates as "sense of place," meaning the way foods and wine express a region's soil, climate, culture, and tradition. We experience the food or beverage based on its geographic identity, for example, Vidalia onions, Vermont maple syrup, Idaho potatoes, Florida oranges, bubbly wine from the Champagne region of France, Mexican tequila, and Egyptian dates. Experiencing place-based foods adds yet another facet of sacredness and wonderment to taking nourishment from earth's bounty—not to mention pleasure! Additionally, a more artisnal approach allows the farmer's product to stand out, garnering a higher price in the marketplace. Because traditional farms are disappearing at an alarming rate, terroir is seen as a way to protect our rural communities; if farmers can earn more money, they're more likely to stay on the land. It's a win-win scenario. Look for artisanal, taste-of-place foods whenever you have a chance.

So go on, be adventurous. Explore! There are so many palate-expanding foods out there. *Remember, beginner's mind;* have an attitude of wonderment, curiosity, and open-mindedness. Really learn how to taste the good life.

Do some reading, investigate herb and spice sites on the Web, ask friends for recommendations, and then write down at least five unfamiliar edibles that you'll purchase on your next grocery-store visit.

PLEASURE-HEALING RITUAL: Wild Foraging for Food

Our ancestors were hunters, gatherers, fishers, and farmers. Food was gathered, raised, or killed and freshly served in relative purity straight from Mother Nature's pantry. With my farming and organic background, I've done my own share of foraging from my community and geographical area. In food foraging, look for wild foods and edibles in your local fields, neighborhood, and backyard. It could be as simple as taking advantage of the pear tree down the way as it drops its fruit in the empty lot. Collect foods that you can easily identify and know are edible, such as apples, plums, citrus, and other tree fruit, as well as blackberries, rose hips, nasturtiums, or violets. This can become quite the hobby, and you'll have lots of fun while you're at it!

To go yet deeper into this practice may take a bit of research and a learning curve, but books and classes abound to further your study. Perhaps your community has a nature center or botanical garden that offers natural-food seminars, where you can learn about gathering and preparing these kinds of foods—from nettle, strawberry leaf, or burdock as tea (they're everywhere in my neighborhood—great blood and kidney detoxifiers!) to dandelion greens (with a bit of goat cheese and walnut oil, or ripe mangoes and honey-lime dressing), fiddlehead ferns, rosehips, cattails, or acorns (acorn pancakes are divine!). With this awareness, perhaps I can inspire you to dabble in your own version of wild foraging from your yard, neighborhood, and parks.

Heighten Your Sense of Taste

Smoking; excess sugar, salt, and fat; and extremes of hot and cold can greatly inhibit your sense of taste. Smoking significantly deadens the sense of smell, such an elemental part of the ability to taste. It also leaves a bitter taste in the mouth that prevents tasting a food's true flavor. Similarly, excess sugar, salt, and fat obscure the natural flavors of food, as does an extremely hot or cold temperature. Ice-cold foods and beverages numb our taste buds, making them less able to discriminate the type and amount of food eaten (they also put out the "digestive fire"; when balanced, our digestive fire allows us to optimally digest or metabolize our food). Scalding heat burns the tongue, inhibiting taste until the damaged taste buds are replaced. Wouldn't you rather roll a sip of beer or hot chocolate around in your mouth to truly taste and enjoy it? Next time, try eating an orange at room temperature, and only heat your soup until *enjoyably* warm to the taste. As you chew, taste the explosion of flavors as you roll the food around in your mouth. Don't be so quick to send it down your throat, because your mouth is where you can truly enjoy the taste. Every second is pure pleasure, so savor the flavor, please!

An Aphrodisiac Banquet: The Love of Food *and* the Food of Love

So many seductive foods beckon us, and we can enjoy them solo or with a significant other. Consider the setting, set the mood, and go for romance—or full-out eroticism. Cardamom, figs, and pomegranates are identified with the feminine, while asparagus, cucumbers, and eggplants are considered masculine. Enjoy it all, feeding both your masculine and feminine sides. Truffles are said to impart a seductive power to those who eat them, while oysters are seen as incredible turn-ons. Other celebrated aphrodisiacs include black beans, blueberries, celery, eggs, dark mushrooms, olives, and ocean and freshwater fish. And let's not forget to include almonds, apricots, bananas, chocolate, dates, figs, honey, licorice, and pine nuts. I suggest having some or all of these foods around to incorporate into your love diet.

MINDFUL EATING

Mindful eating is a practice similar to meditation, prayer, or physical activity. First and foremost, you have to devote yourself to eating mindfully, beginning with your intention. Becoming mindful of the nourishment we enjoy, on all levels, makes it much easier to make healthy food selections, eat reasonable portions, and truly enjoy eating rather than simply fill our tummies. Naturally, this not only applies to the actual food that we put on our plates but also to the way we digest it. Rethink your definition of digestion as more than the process by which you convert food into simpler chemical compounds for assimilation by the body. Broaden the meaning to include not only the food you eat but also your attitude as you eat it.

We digest, metabolize, and assimilate all of life's experiences into who we are, into our mind-body physiology. Because eating is one of these experiences, it should be one of life's greatest pleasures. Eating with awareness of, and appreciation for, the nourishment you take in increases your ability to assimilate nutrients. The opposite is also true: eating when you're stressed out, rushed, or in a dark mood makes your digestive system function far less efficiently. How often have you had heartburn, gastrointestinal upset, bloating, or general malaise after a particularly heavy, unhealthy meal?

As we return to seeing eating as a sacred ritual and an agricultural act, pure goodness from the earth, a major shift happens in our attitude. Eating well becomes a celebration.

Take Your Time

It takes a full twenty minutes for your brain to register satiety. Eating too quickly and gorging on your food dramatically increases your caloric intake per sitting, because you're eating way more than your body needs. When you "stuff and swallow," you miss 90 percent of the taste of the foods you eat, and also severely compromise your digestive and overall metabolic processing of your food. Many of us can use a gentle reminder to take a mindfulness-based approach to eating. A yogi taught me, "Drink your food, and eat your drink," thoroughly chewing every bite of food before swallowing. Digestion begins in our mouths with the release of saliva and the mastication of our food. Eat with full awareness and appreciation for the nourishment you're taking in. Instead of going on restrictive diets that make you feel deprived, guilty, and stressed, enjoy your beloved delicacies more slowly and in smaller amounts. You'll automatically eat less and enjoy more. Remember, you're not just feeding your taste buds; let food nourish all your senses. The more you engage with the aromas, textures, colors, and even the sounds of eating, the more deeply the food will satisfy you and the less likely you'll be to overindulge.

The spa community and yours truly are huge proponents of the Slow Food international movement, a nonprofit organization with over eighty thousand members worldwide (see www.slowfood.com) whose aim is to protect the pleasures of the table from the homogenization of modern fast food and high-paced life. According to the Slow Food movement, savoring a wide variety of foods is key to "eco-gastronomical" well-being. Slow foodists believe we've become so consumed by the need for speed and efficiency that we've lost the ability to appreciate the finer things in life. If you're into food prepared the old-fashioned way and in a sustainable fashion, add slow foods to your daily menu for a more vibrant palate.

PLEASURE-HEALING RITUAL: An Eating Meditation

To learn the fine art of eating with spirit, here's how to take your next meal: Settle yourself into a comfortable spot with your food, a place where you won't be distracted. No TV! Give your full attention to every facet of the eating experience.

Give thanks for every person and circumstance that brought this food to you: the farmer who nurtured the soil and planted the seeds; the sun's life-giving warmth and energy that helped the food grow; all those who helped harvest, process, and transport it to your grocer or farmers' market. If you're eating animal foods, be especially thankful that this animal gave his life to help you sustain yours. Don't forget to give thanks for whoever lovingly prepared the food, including yourself, if you prepared it! Perhaps say grace; for example, "Bless this food before me, and all those who brought it to my table."

Now look closely at the food. Become intimate with its shape, form, and texture. Use all your senses, and take in the colors. Touch the food, if possible. Perhaps bring it to your nose. Smell the aromas. Let the food rest for a moment on your lips. Can you feel the saliva already beginning to flow in your mouth? You should! All these sensory steps enact the digestive process.

After putting a small amount of food into your mouth, chew thoroughly, feeling how your jaw moves and tasting the explosion of flavors. Exercise every one of those ten thousand taste buds across the broad expanse of your tongue. Experience the subtle nuances of all six tastes in your food choices: sweet, sour, salty, pungent, bitter, and astringent.

After you've thoroughly chewed the food, mentally follow it down your esophagus and into your stomach. Pay attention to any sensations in your stomach. Stay connected to mindfulness with every bite of your meal if possible. If you're using utensils, remind yourself to mindfully put them down between bites. Don't gulp beverages during this eating meditation. Drinking liquids at a meal isn't necessary when you thoroughly chew your food. As you continue relishing each bite, you'll begin to feel the sensation of fullness.

After finishing your meal, sit for a few moments, breathing smoothly and naturally. Give thanks again for the food and its life-giving sustenance. After a few reflective moments, get up and go for a brief walk; five to ten minutes will do. This will enhance the digestive process even further.

Now think back over the entire process. Did you feel as if you were in super-duper slow motion? Great! This is how we were meant to take in nourishment. If you do nothing other than eat mindfully, you'll not only maintain or lose weight but also trans-form the entire eating experience into a joyful celebration or ritual. Your relationship to food will change forever.

Prepare for Ecstasy

Besides making a spiritual connection through mindful eating, you can engage with a mystical level of higher consciousness through food preparation. When making a meal or snack, prepare every morsel with as much love and compassion as possible. When my beloved husband James cooks our meals (he's a classically trained French chef—I know, I know, I'm a very fortunate woman!), he does so with the very best energy possible. The food is filled with love and compassion, not only for its content and origin but also for the process of taking in the most wholesome and organic foods possible. James is in a state of flow as he chops, dices, mixes, marinates, adds spices and herbs, makes sauces, bakes, and steams. Then, with great anticipation and gratitude, we joyfully sit down to this food feast. Another part of the ritual is that we open a bottle of fine wine from James's wine cellar to sip during our flavorful repast. When you learn to cook with care and reverence, you, too, will discover that food, body, and nature are the same entity. Our bodily flesh is made from the flesh of our healthful food, which is living, breathing tissue. Just imagine this! The energy and intelligence from our food becomes the energy and intelligence of our mind-body physiology.

Taking the Waters

After oxygen, water's the second most important substance to sustain life. And it's the most abundant substance in the body. This vital liquid accounts for around 80 percent of the body's weight; our muscles are 75 percent water, and our blood is 90 percent water. Water's crucial for carrying out almost every bodily function, including transporting nutrients throughout the body and removing metabolic waste from our cells. Water oxygenates our blood and increases our energy levels, and also plays a major role in regulating normal elimination, a vital form of detoxification.

It's important to drink purified or filtered water. Try your best to minimize ice-cold water or beverages, because they diminish the "digestive fire," which optimizes metabolism of food. As mentioned previously, excessively cold drinks can also numb the taste buds, decreasing their ability to discriminate how much and what's being eaten, and lessening our overall enjoyment of food.

Consider your hydration quota both at home and work. If it's not provided at work, bring a supply of your own filtered water from home in a large glass jar. Tossing in some fruit imparts a wonderful flavor; try sliced oranges, lemons, limes, kiwi, cucumber, or berries. Drink sparkling or mineral water instead of soda. Also consider hot or cold herbal teas.

When we first start paying attention to our water intake, sometimes we notice how amazingly little we actually consume. Again, remember sweet mindfulness. Make yourself accountable until water consumption becomes a glorious habit. Take your journal and note how much you sip throughout the course of the day, and continue doing so for one week. At the end of each day, add up the ounces. Do you come up with a minimum of sixty-four ounces? You simply won't believe how great this makes you feel!

PLEASURE-HEALING RITUAL: The Art, Celebration, and Pleasure of Tea Time

While we're on the subject of mindful sipping, let me share the virtues of taking tea, the world's most prized elixir and the most consumed beverage on the planet, second only to water. More than a drink, it's a deep social and cultural ritual, a pause in the day, a health-giving infusion. An ancient Japanese proverb says, "If a man has no tea in him, he is incapable of understanding truth and beauty." Indeed, the tea ritual, with its focus on gentleness, hospitality, and spending quiet time together, has come to symbolize enlightened spiritual vision. You can imbibe black, green, oolong, or herbal teas. Whether a milky Darjeeling (lovely with a piece of dark chocolate after dinner!); a strong, emerald matcha; a delicate oolong jasmine; or perhaps one of many herbal infusions, such as a sweet, red rooibos, a world of teas is available for our healing, meditative pleasure. And healing, they are; drinking tea has many health benefits, not least of which are enhanced digestion, lowered cholesterol, and reduced risk of cancer. You can appreciate tea culture in the surging tea-room scene, the spa tea ceremony, or your own afternoon or after-dinner tea time at home. Taking tea ever invites us to focus our minds, and creates an atmosphere of contemplative calm.

Believed to have originated in China over five thousand years ago, tea is still treated with immense reverence in the East. When you realize the care that goes into harvesting, preparing, and serving a cup of the brew—the hand-plucked leaves, the pure water, the exacting temperature and timing for brewing, the type of cup, and the "tea mind" with which it's enjoyed—you really do get the magic. For instance, in the traditional Japanese ceremony, the sensual brush of the textured cup against your lips is almost as important as the taste of the tea itself.

Whether a traditional Eastern approach or today's Western versions of enjoying tea, you can appreciate that the taking of tea is a form of gratifying, enlightening, and uplifting meditation—so much so, that who of us wouldn't want to make it a daily happening! You make it so with your intention.

THE INCREDIBLE HEALING POWER OF FOOD

Hippocrates said, "Let food be your medicine, and medicine be your food," which has never been more relevant than today, since new and powerful compounds within whole foods are being uncovered that are truly medicinal in their actions. A diet containing five servings of such powerhouse foods as vegetables, fruits, and whole grains a day may prevent well over 20 percent of all cancers, including colon, stomach, lung, esophagus, breast, bladder, pancreas, and prostate. These miracles from nature contain powerful cancer fighters called *antioxidants*, which stabilize free radicals and halt cellular damage. Free radicals are harmful, reactive molecules that help set the stage for major chronic diseases, such as cancer and accelerated aging. Most abundant in organically grown plants, some of the most powerful antioxidants include vitamins A or beta-carotene (a precursor to vitamin A), C, E, the B's, and that powerhouse mineral selenium.

Begin listening to your inner wisdom today, and fight the urge to consume larger amounts of saturated and trans fats, sugar, salt, and refined carbs. Get rid of the ersatz foods in your kitchen: anything processed, fat free, artificially sweetened, chemically enhanced, or otherwise manipulated. Stock up on rich, flavorful, whole foods, organic whenever possible, and begin to really nourish your mind and body. Teach yourself to truly relish the delicious, natural flavors of life. Eat a fresh carrot and savor the sublime sweetness. Try your whole-grain cereal without added sugar, and appreciate the grain's natural sweetness. Eat your watermelon without salt and your grapefruit without sugar. Spritz with a lemon or lime slice first, so you can cut back on the dressing on your salad or butter on your steamed veggies. Instead of butter's saturated fat, dribble on a bit of organic olive, peanut, rice-bran, grapeseed, or sesame oil. Infuse these oils with herbs and spices. In fact, instead of reaching for the salt or sugar, use herbs and spices in all your favorite foods. Really tasting the fresh, delectable, pungent flavors will eventually retrain your taste buds to enjoy the natural flavor and goodness of food.

FOOD FOR THOUGHT

The keys to healthful eating couldn't be simpler: mindfulness, moderation, and common sense; on the most practical level, calories in, calories out. Yes, this will involve daily consideration, but we're talking about our health and longevity here, right? Be super choosy about the foods you eat, not just for a couple of weeks or months but for the rest of your life.

Take time to reflect on your eating habits. Consider a typical day, at home and at work. If you'd like to change your eating habits, keeping a journal of your thoughts and experiences around eating can help disconnect you from any unhealthy urges. Also consider seeing a nutritionist.

Eat in a quiet, settled environment. Don't eat when you're emotionally overwrought. Before you eat, do some deep breathing to quiet down your overactive mind.

Eat only when hungry. Listen to your appetite.

Eat at a comfortable pace. Fully chew each bite of food, all the while staying conscious of the process. The digestive process begins in the mouth.

Don't overeat. Leave a portion of your stomach empty to aid the digestive process.

Sit quietly for a few minutes after eating. Focus on the sensations in your body. Then go for a short walk to aid the digestive process.

Listen to your body and your moods. Witness how your body reacts to your food choices, and modulate accordingly.

It's never too late to change your eating habits and begin treating yourself to wholesome, nutritious, *and* delicious food. Know that a healthy diet does beautiful things not only for your body's inside (immune system and energy level) but also for your outer beauty (skin, hair, and nails), as well as your attitude (optimistic, resilient, and compassionate). You'll feel vibrantly alive, function at your highest physical, mental, creative, and emotional levels and set the best possible example for all those in your sphere of influence. Become obsessive about it. Trust me when I tell you that eating healthfully and joyfully is a wonderful obsession to have. Now go munch on some fresh green beans with a drizzle of basil-infused olive oil, and enjoy life!

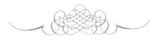

CHAPTER 6

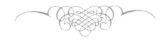

MINDFULNESS IN MOTION

You have to stay in shape. My grandmother—she started walking five miles a day when she was sixty. She's ninety-seven today and we don't know where the hell she is.

—ELLEN DEGENERES

Our bodies love to move! Every minute you devote to physical activity is a blessing for your body, mind, and soul. Along with proper nutrition, it's one of the greatest healers. Physical activity is not only vital to our well-being, it's also one of the most powerful beautifiers there is, creating inner *and* outer beauty. Think about how you feel *and* look after any physical activity. Look in the mirror after your lunchtime walk, and see an inviting smile replace that mid-morning harried scowl. How beautiful is that? And how about your skin's natural luminescence after a thirty-minute workout? No amount of blush can produce such a radiant glow! As an expression of spirit, your body is most blissful when it moves with the life force flowing through it, whether you're at work or at play.

We all know the importance of physical activity. Yet, many choose not to engage in even the most minimal amount of daily activity necessary for health. Sufficient exercise is one of the foremost critical ingredients for living a vibrant, joyful life, and so many place it at the bottom of the priority list. Perhaps this is due to the time we live in, where many feel spiritually deprived; when we're disconnected from our inner sense, lethargy and inertia set it. This is another area where sweet mindfulness comes into "play."

Spirit loves to play! Connecting to spirit makes you an energetic bundle of joy, enthusiasm, and effervescence. I know how good my daily "play" makes me feel in body, mind, and mood. Why not see all of our daily movement activities as play?

MAKING THE CONNECTION: WHY MOVEMENT MATTERS

Now for a bit of the philosophical stuff: movement connects intention to action. When we're sedentary, our intentions become disconnected from our actions. We can have the best intentions, but our movement deficit prevents us from acting on them. It's then, in this state of inactivity, that we risk losing one of our most precious gifts: spontaneity. This loss makes it difficult to engage joyfully and passionately in any effort toward fulfillment of our goals.

Moreover, this chasm, or disconnect, between thought and action can result in inertia and profound fatigue. It sounds illogical that nonmovement creates fatigue, but it's a fact. Exercise, healing movement, play—the regular, deliberate, and pleasurable physical movement of the body—can stave off this inertia.

If we forsake regular physical movement and disconnect our intentions from our actions, depression, or at least some aspects of this debilitating mental illness, becomes a real possibility. An old saying comes to mind: "The mind is willing, but the body is not." When this happens, we tend to give up, making ourselves prime targets for melancholy or even despondency.

What's more, without spontaneity and conscious movement, daily tensions can gain the upper hand, lacing the body and psyche in a straightjacket of sorts. The emotional body is not separate from the physical body. With tension, our bodies start to "grip," to clench and tighten up. Fascia, the connective tissue that surrounds and encases our muscles, can form harmful holding patterns. Consider the hurts, strains, and sprains we experience when we become passive about our activity or our life-force energy. Everything becomes such an effort. Simply standing up from the couch can be a strain for the couch potato. For anyone who is physically inactive and rigid, merely walking across the room could produce an ankle blowout. If you're weak, inflexible, and unfit, bending over to tie your shoes or pick up your child could easily throw out your lower back.

There are so many people currently wearing this metaphoric straightjacket that many antidotes are prescribed and have been developed for it. Naturally, meditation, in all its forms, is numero uno. When we become exquisitely present, we automatically know that movement is an absolute in our day-to-day lives. Yoga, including pranayama, or healing breath work, is a champion at releasing mental and bodily tension. Other remedies include bodywork, such as myofascial release (*myo* means "muscle," and *fascial* means "fascia"), which was created specifically to disengage these fixed (and for some, long-held) patterns in the fascia. Rolfing is another well-known approach. Neurostructural Integration Technique (NST) can also be quite helpful, because it not only releases held patterns but also rebalances the body's energy circuits. These are but a few remedies.

If left unattended, physical or mental stress begins to prevent free-flowing movement into new thought processes and positions. The restriction in the body feeds restriction in the mind, and vice versa, resulting in quite the feedback loop and not a pleasurable one! Our minds start to establish parameters beyond which we're not allowed to move, so that "I can't do that" becomes our new reality. Range of motion and flexibility in body *and* mind are drastically reduced so that only certain movements and habits are permitted. Over time, we can suffer debilitating physical and emotional diseases. Regular free-flowing movement releases you from this type of stranglehold. So, get moving, and find out how movement affects every facet of your being. The expansiveness you'll feel will be awe inspiring. Pleasurable movement is a primary way to ignite, renew, or maintain the vital link between our intentions and our actions, reconnecting us with our spontaneous and joyful love of life. What a beautiful and positive feedback loop this is!

As a mind-body health educator, massage therapist, personal trainer, and triathlete, one of my strongest desires is to have the persuasive power or eloquence to convince everyone I meet of the importance of moving the body—abundantly. Physical activity has such tremendous healing powers and restorative effects. The best part is that you can begin this process of getting physical (and profoundly change your mind-body health for the better) wherever you are today, and steadily progress toward your optimal fitness, whatever your age, weight, gender, or present conditioning.

JUST DO IT!

As in any life-affirming practice, the key is psyching ourselves to "just do it." Many look for inspiration to become active. It's often easier to become the couch potato in our convenience-oriented world, where technology and machines in the form of remote controls, leaf blowers, drive-up windows, and the like have streamlined our lives while rendering our bodies less mobile. In addition, work sites and urban areas have been designed to minimize walking while increasing commercial convenience. We've engineered movement right out of our lives! Think of ways you can weave it into your life wherever you can as "stealth" exercise. I strongly encourage you to rethink all the movements you make during the day, and try to use the more physical approach whenever possible. Although, socioculturally we've stacked the deck against devoting ourselves to consistent daily exercise, I'm certain your ingenuity can shine a light on the path of least resistance toward optimal daily movement. Each and every one of us must simply set this intention. Our lives might just depend on it. Not one of us would want a catastrophic illness to be our motivation to become physically active. Let's all think of physical activity as a lifelong prescription for health and longevity.

LET'S GET PHYSICAL

Physical activity includes cardiovascular, flexibility, and strengthening activities. Try to create a balance of these three types of activity in your daily movement. And please do enjoy the process! Imagine your body pumping out those mood-enhancing, joy-inducing, pain-relieving endorphins. Imagine supporting your heart, the busiest muscle in your body. Imagine fueling your body and mind with energy, shoring up your metabolism, powering up your immunity, shifting your shape, and so much more. Coming from a place of mental focus (read: mindfulness) greatly enhances the benefits of your activity.

Cardiovascular activity improves the body's capacity to use fuel and oxygen, and greatly enhances your heart health, immune system, endurance, longevity, and overall quality of life. It's well known for its stress-reducing benefit. Every hour of activity can provide a two-hour increase in life span. Consider brisk walking; jogging; swimming; biking; dancing; jumping rope; or doing power yoga, pilates, or Nia (a loosely choreographed form of dance integrating martial and healing arts, that allows the body's wisdom to express itself in free-flowing and joyful movement).

Flexibility exercises are great for easing physical tension; improving range of motion and agility; and helping connect body, mind, and spirit. Concentrating on your breathing during these activities brings you face-to-face with your energy source. Try yoga, tai chi, pilates, and Nia.

Strengthening or weight-bearing activities enhance your power, endurance, balance, and coordination. Along with the aesthetic benefits (such as toned muscles and cellulite reduction), your body will also build bones and muscle, boosting your metabolic furnace and efficiently burning fat. You can use free weights, machines, or resistance bands, as well as perform weight-bearing activities such as walking, yoga, or pilates (one of my all-time favorites for developing core strength).

Try to fit a balance of all three types of activities into your day.

FIVE EASY PIECES

Mark Twain once said, "Oh, I get the urge to exercise every now and then, but I just lay down 'til it goes away." Now, you may find this amusing, as did I, but in reality, I know that you'll find physical exercise far more entertaining. In other words, you'll enjoy the way physical activity helps balance your mind-body physiology. It feels so good; it feels so right; it's what our bodies are meant to do. There are some species that have flat or immovable facets or joints. Not us; we have synovial, or movable, joints: gliding, ball and socket, hinge, and so on. We're meant to move our bodies, and bodies in motion tend to stay in motion. Keep yours moving. There's nothing more freeing than movement coupled with the exhilaration of deep breathing. To help you discover this joy, I offer five easy steps: (1) change your mind-set, (2) find time for movement, (3) visualize yourself as fit in the future, (4) focus on the astonishing benefits, and (5) be aware that exercise enhances the mood.

Change Your Mind-Set

Your first step toward true enjoyment of physical activity is to change your mind-set. Physical activity is a "get to," not a "have to." Reframing movement in this way nurtures an appreciation and, ultimately, a love of it! I've personally worked with the physically disabled, so trust me when I say that any one of them would give anything to be able to get up and go for a walk. God forbid, but if you were paralyzed tomorrow and no longer able to move, it would be your greatest desire to do so. This may sound a bit harsh, but because I've provided yoga therapy for stroke-recovery and wheelchair-bound patients, this awareness is at the top of my mind. This awareness gives me a much-needed kick-start whenever I'm waffling about exercising! Create a shift in your perception, your awareness. Instead of taking your ability to move for granted, cherish it. Become fiercely devoted to your love of exercise, and don't let up. Too many of us view exercise as drudgery, something to ignore altogether or get through as quickly as possible as if it were punishment. Instead, why not see it as a delectable dessert? See healing movement as a gift, not a chore. It's such a joy to move your body and get your endorphins flowing. See movement as an opportunity to stretch yourself in every direction: physically, mentally, and spiritually.

Fit for Fun

I suggest you conjure up beginner's mind, and see any form of movement, whether free form or structured, as "child's play." Take the work out of "workout," and put more play in your day. View any physical activity with a sense of wonderment and wide-eyed delight. See to it that you're one of the lucky ones who's in on the secret of fitness as fun and decadent delight. This mind-set helps us enjoy the organic pleasure, the sheer joy, of movement. We're not moving because we have to but because it's so much fun! What a shame we have to grow up! When we were babies, we instinctively sat straight, and ate just until we were full. As toddlers, we could never sit still; we danced, shook, and shimmied, letting our limbs move freely about. Walking would never do when there was running to be done, and stairs were mountains to be climbed and explored. Did our tummies stick out when we were children? Who remembers? There was too much fun to be had to worry about such things. And then we grew up, and of all the things we've "forgotten," our relationship with our natural bodies is perhaps the most tragic. When did tearing around stop being fun? When bits of us started to wobble, when our lungs could no longer keep up with our intentions, or when moving became another chore to schedule into our day. Well, I say you can recapture this magic, this playfulness. Intention, visualization, and affirmation will get you there. Bring your sense of play into your physical activities, whatever they are. There are so many pleasurable things to do with your body: mountain climbing, outward-bound adventures, canoeing the local waterways, walking labyrinths! Remember the *Sex and the City* episode highlighting the trapeze arts? Would that be called "sexercise"? Ooh-la-la! Or how about a belly-dancing class? If ever there was a dance of the goddess! So let the games begin!

Pleasure-Healing Ritual: Rhythm Games

Remember those fun rhythm games you played as a child? Hopscotch, jacks, jump rope, hula hoop, paddleball. And let's not forget the trampoline, even in today's incarnation: the mini trampoline. These games required skill and concentration but also, and perhaps more important, a sense of rhythm and coordination. You can revisit any of these games today for a physical-activity jump start, a good workout, and certainly a cheap thrill!

Once mastered, games such as jump rope and hula hoop (called "hooping" these days) improve your endurance and flexibility while raising your heartbeat. More than just kids' toys, jacks and paddleball also reinforce fitness-related benefits such as timing and rhythm, speed and agility. The mini trampoline affords a culmination of aerobic, dance, and sport-specific movements that literally can kick your butt but are low impact on your joints.

Hooping is one of my favorites. You get a great cardiovascular workout, strengthening every major muscle group and increasing flexibility in every major joint region. I call it a "gateway" activity, because it opens the door to a more well-rounded approach to health, encouraging us to pursue other avenues to physical wellness, such as yoga and dance classes. My big red hula hoop is always at the ready; it gives me the greatest workout and many laughs in my backyard, where my pooches go bananas over this fun oddity I gyrate with. The hoop has many moves to learn, such as balancing it, building steady momentum, recovering it, and doing basic side-to-side steps and full rotations. My sore abs and arms speak to hooping's physical benefits, so it's easy to see how regular practice can carve out a trim and defined waist, a tight midsection, and better flexibility. What ultimately drew me to hooping was the fun factor. Though it conjures up memories of childhood play, hooping isn't just for the under-twelve set. It's about dance, coordination, strength building, movement, and even sensuality—and it's criminally entertaining, to boot!

Find Time

The second step many of us need to take before we can truly learn to enjoy physical activity is to find time. This may be a biggie for some of you—and a primary reason for not exercising. But truly, this is about prioritizing our lives and goals. Put making time for movement right up there at the very top of the list with spiritual development, stress management, and a healthful diet. If you make a commitment to just start some form of physical activity, you'll begin to experience dramatic change so that movement naturally becomes a higher priority. You may even be amazed at how many minutes you find for a little stretching here and a little walking there—and a bit here and there do count. Ten minutes of running in the morning on your treadmill or outdoors, a brisk walk after lunch and dinner (so good for optimizing the digestion), a few yoga stretches at intervals throughout the day, perhaps a few more when you get home at night—all do cumulative good, and all count.

If you don't like structured physical activity, be creative. Put on some great, driving music, and dance free-form in your living room. Wash the kitchen floor to a beat. If your passion is shopping, walk the entire mall (twice!) before buying that yummy new jacket. See raking leaves as Zen time. If budget, health-club accessibility, or neighborhood safety are considerations for you, consider borrowing exercise, yoga, pilates, dance, or one of the many other physical-activity DVDs or videos from your local library or video-rental store. Also, many communities and park districts have a gym or weight room that you can use free of charge. My mother always said, "Where there's a will, there's a way." Amen to that. Here's my favorite: "If we can fly people to the moon, we can do this!" Ultimately, it's about mind over matter.

Now that you know how good exercise is for you, let me steer you toward a few vital tools that can actualize introspection and attitudinal changes.

Visualize Yourself as Fit in the Future

The third step is to use your visualization skills to imagine yourself in all the stages of life that lie before you. Anyone, at any age, can visualize and affirm his or her desire to play and be fit. We all have the ability to imagine ourselves in the best of circumstances; perhaps you can visualize yourself at sixty, seventy, or even eighty, still taking that early-morning swim, pedaling to the marketplace, or briskly walking a few miles each morning. Keep the positive affirmations going full-throttle. As you engage your body and mind, whatever the activity, say to yourself, "Every day, in every way, I'm getting better and better." See how healthy, vigorous, mentally sharp, and energetic you feel as you enjoy every moment of every day. Contrast this with an image of yourself as a potentially bedridden, overweight, and constantly fatigued elder who truly feels old. No, you say? You can't or won't imagine this miserable scenario? Okay then, stick with the beautiful, healthy visual. It just might inspire you to begin or maintain your dedication to a daily regimen of physical activity. Visualization and positive affirmation are ever so powerful at manifesting our desires. Put your intention out there into the universe. With great optimism and commitment, begin devoting time daily to movement activities. Visualize how your mind and body are transforming for the better with each moment of movement. Every day, affirm your devotion to your practice. Remember, it takes thirty days to instill a new habit. As you integrate "playtime" into your daily routine, schedule and mark such time on each day of your calendar. Write, "I did it!" or draw a red heart. I promise you'll find it much easier to keep going. You're in the process of changing your lifestyle and transforming your core being for the rest of your life. This is fantastic stuff!

Focus on the Astonishing Benefits

The fourth step to learning to love physical activity is to focus on the benefits of movement; once you finish reading this section, you'll have intrinsic knowledge. You'll understand how regular exercise benefits every physical and mental process. On a sweeping level, it enhances our energy and stamina levels, a big issue for many of us. Exercising regularly also provides a powerful boost to the immune system, which is absolutely essential in this day and age of many mental, emotional, and physical stressors, including environmental toxins. Just for a moment, consider how many daily interactions you have with others. We're afloat in a sea of bacteria, and the healthiest of immune systems is our number-one safety net against a barrage of potential assaults to our mind-body physiology. Healing movement can make you stronger and more resilient than you could ever imagine.

Moving on to specifics, the entire body benefits from regular movement. Regular, consistent physical activity benefits the heart and blood vessels, musculoskeletal system, and respiration, our ability to take deep diaphragmatic breaths. Improved cardiovascular and respiratory function enhances transport of oxygen and nutrients to every cell in the body, increases HDL (the good cholesterol), and reduces the risk of adult-onset diabetes. It's also key to managing or reducing weight and body fat. Regular physical activity enhances all of our gastrointestinal processes—digestion, absorption, and elimination—moving carbon dioxide and waste products from the body tissues into the bloodstream and then to the eliminative organs, whether through breathing, perspiration, urination, or bowel movements. Maybe that's why it cuts the risk of colon cancer in half, and lowers cancer rates in general. Metabolic wastes and lactic acid collect in our bodies when we stop moving, which further supports the claim that regular exercise can be one of the most powerful rituals for detoxification.

In this stressful day and age, we need to protect and support all of the body's natural and constant detoxification processes to reduce the buildup of toxins. How comforting it is to know that we can enhance the detox process through consistent physical activity.

Mood Enhancement, Anyone?

Had a bad day? Here's your fifth and final reason to love exercise! Physical activity is one of the absolute-best stress busters and mood enhancers. It constructively counters cortisol (a primary stress hormone) and other fight-or-flight hormones released during high-stress situations. In addition, regular exercisers have higher self-esteem and a generally happier outlook. Have you heard of the "runner's high"? This occurs, because exercise triggers release of endorphins, inducing a feeling of exhilaration. The resulting mood elevation lasts from 90 to 120 minutes after an exercise session, and the increase in basal metabolic rate hums on well past that. In addition, it's my understanding that well-known physician Andrew Weil, MD, frequently prescribes aerobic exercise as a safe and effective treatment for depression, because exercise stimulates the release of endorphins, which are a class of internal antidepressants created in the brain. Exercise both treats and prevents depression in susceptible individuals. Dr. Weil recommends forty-five minutes of sustained aerobic activity an average of five days a week, though any activity that raises your heart rate and gets you breathing fast will help, for example, fast or uphill walking.

From your mood to your metabolism, your heart to your immune system, your muscles to your bones, exercise is the cat's meow. Here are some more-personal reasons why I love physical activity: it gets me out of the house and into nature, where I disengage from the world of machines and expose myself to the sun, sky, and wind. I can walk in the natural light and enjoy the sights, sounds, and smells that awaken me to the extraordinary beauty around me! I meet great people and keep up on the happenings in my neighborhood. Exercise gives me something interesting to talk about and helps me sleep. Oh, and my poochies love their walk! Look for reasons unique to you, and treasure them! And let's not forget, there's nothing sexier than someone who takes good care of his or her body and mind through consistent physical activity! It's the ultimate turn-on—and head turner! Reflect on this for a moment. Regular movement will make you feel and appear vital, robust, strong, *and* young, whatever your age.

Healing Movement (or "Playtime") Journal

Open your notebook or journal and answer the following questions. Feel free to add your own spontaneous thoughts. Then go take a walk!

1. What are your exercise habits? Describe them in terms of intensity, frequency, and duration.

2. How often do you put in a little extra physical-activity time, and what form does it take? For example, do you take the stairs instead of the elevator? Do you ever park in the farthest space or down the side street and then walk to your destination, be it work, a store, or the doctor's office?

3. Do you go by foot instead of car when running neighborhood errands?

4. What physical activities do you enjoy most?

5. Where are some lovely places to enjoy walking, biking, jogging, or in-line skating?

6. What inspires you to get up and get going? Perhaps make this a frequently used visualization or positive affirmation.

7. What incentives or rewards might help you maintain a regular physical-activity regime? (Make these incentives realistic, and if you do get up and go, don't forget to give yourself the promised reward!)

8. Do you have buddies who might enjoy taking brisk walks with you?

9. List other ideas that could inspire you to move your body.

Let's enjoy some practices now, shall we? Mindful, or serenity-generating, movement activities are very popular right now. Spa wisdom, the world's spiritual awakening, and the aging baby-boomer population have had a great impact on this trend. Yoga, tai chi, pilates, and the many other relaxation workouts out there are all about slowing down and finding balance. You can think of them as "total awareness" workouts or stress-free fitness activities.

POSTURE PERFECT

Let's begin at the beginning, by talking about our posture, or perhaps more accurately, postural derangement. More people are experiencing severe back issues that they believe require serious intervention when simple postural alignment might help. Most of us are born with healthy spines, but more than half of all adults develop back problems by age thirty. Lower-back pain is second only to the common cold as the major cause of absenteeism from work, costing upwards of seventy billion dollars a year in the United States alone. Yet, you only have to observe a young child sitting on the floor with a perfectly balanced back or visit India or Africa and notice the old women squatting on their heels to know that it's possible to have a perfectly easy, natural, and pain-free relationship with your spine. Its roots in Western civilization (where our modern lifestyle causes much of our dysfunction), back pain is not so common in China, where large numbers of the population practice gentle, rhythmic tai chi in the parks in the morning, and in Muslim countries, where people's spines ritually bend and stretch in worship up to five times a day.

Are your lower-back muscles tight and tense? Do you regularly experience muscle spasms? Do you walk around with your shoulders rolled forward and hoisted up somewhere near your ears? Poor posture affects our health on every level, triggering a cascade of tiny structural changes throughout the body that have painful consequences. The shoulders, neck, and head push forward; and the pelvis tilts and shifts the spine, putting added pressure on muscles and joints. When combined, these habits distort and compress the spine.

When the spine is out of balance, the rest of the body repatterns itself to compensate. Some muscles tighten up and shorten, while others become overstretched and weak. Certain muscles work overtime to stabilize the body, and over time this repatterning becomes habitual, which is when true imbalances set in, causing pain and injury. Neurological problems result as well, given that the spinal cord houses the central nervous system. On an energetic level, poor posture greatly depletes our energy. When your shoulders consistently hunch forward so that your rib cage collapses over your solar plexus, you can't breathe optimally. You can't effectively exhale tension.

PLEASURE-HEALING RITUAL: Yoga's Tadasana or Mountain Pose

What better way to practice postural, or spinal, alignment than with *tadasana* or mountain pose. This posture will bring you immediate expansiveness, opening, and release. It also develops strength and agility in the mind and body, and stretches and aligns the spine, enhancing energy flow. A healthy spine is a column of flowing biological energy, allowing us to breathe more effectively, which delivers oxygenated blood throughout the body and especially to the brain:

1. Breathe smoothly and deeply, using your diaphragm.

2. Stand with your feet under your hips. Imagine that the soles of your feet are grounded into the earth. Lift your toes and separate them as if you're trying to see

119

space between them. Now plant them down into the earth. Feel the connection to the earth's energy.

3. Draw your head back and stack it over your shoulders. Stand tall, reaching the crown of your head toward the sky.

4. Roll your shoulders back and down, moving the shoulder blades toward each other. Feel how this opens the heart center. Relish it!

5. Gently draw your tailbone down toward the earth, which draws the lower abs inward. This is a highly desirable "neutral spine" position not only practiced in yoga sessions but also useful in your work and play activities.

6. As you reach your crown toward the heavens and your tailbone into the earth, you're nurturing and decompressing the spine. Take as many breaths as you have time for while in this position.

Eventually you'll want to maintain this posture all the time. This type of posture not only exudes poise, strength, and self-confidence but also makes you look taller and slimmer—guaranteed.

Good posture takes awareness and vigilance, so begin today to witness your posture. Be sure to get enough regular physical activity to stretch and lengthen your spine, loosen up tight hip muscles, and strengthen abdominal muscles to take the load off your back. Consider regular yoga practice and pilates. Yoga renders the entire body more flexible, tones muscles, and releases tension, while pilates not only boosts your heart rate but also isolates, strengthens, tones, and releases muscles, as well as firms and tightens the abdominals (important for healthy spinal alignment and balance).

Discussing good posture includes mentioning shoes. In my business, I see it all, including poor footwear choices, such as an ill fit, high heels, and narrow, pointy toes. Along with blisters, bunions, plantar fasciitis, bone spurs, and a host of other foot problems, an unhealthy and habitual repatterning of the musculoskeletal system will happen, perhaps not today, this week, or this month, but trust that, if you wear unhealthy shoes, you'll have to eventually seek medical treatment for myriad bodily aches and pains. High heels totally change the mechanics of how you walk and stand. Those who often wear high heels generally have shortened, tight Achilles tendons. Your legs and lower back are meant to work together as one seamless unit, but foot problems limit your ability to walk fluidly, forcing other muscles to pick up the slack and causing repetitive strain on your lower back. High heels also throw off your center of gravity, creating an unnatural curve (*lordosis*) in the lower back that can become very painful. So opt for round or square toed shoes and under-two-inch heels. Your spinal health and optimal well-being depend on it!

Moving onward to mindful-movement activities, let's begin with the most accessible for us all, mindful walking. I'm a huge champion of walking. And when imbued with your full presence, you can certainly make this activity one of pure healing pleasure.

121

PLEASURE-HEALING RITUAL: Enlightened Walking

It's said, "Wherever you go, there you are"—if you're present, that is! Oh sure, we may be physically present, but we're mentally and emotionally absent. Walking is a great activity to practice being fully present—body, mind, and soul. Enlightened walking? You bet! When we walk, we can be totally engaged, paying attention to every step, breath, and sensation. The cadence of your walk and your breath can become a form of meditation that lulls and comforts you into serene repose.

Walking is a primordial exercise. It's widely accessible, doesn't need any special equipment, and brings us out into the neighborhood and nature. Be exquisitely present when you walk! Free your mind from distractions, and be in the moment. Wake up to the extraordinary beauty around you! Enjoy the sights, sounds, and aromas. And as you expose yourself to the sun, skies, and wind, take time to thank Mother Earth for all she does to nurture us. Witness your senses awakening without the burden of thought or a running commentary in your mind. Keep your mind open and expansive. Your walk can include a state of gratitude, with lots of positive self-talk, or you can concentrate on body mechanics as you walk: the powerful swing of your arms; the way you lift your foot, swing it, and place it down (heel to toe); and the way your breathing feels as your pace changes. I have a dialogue with myself as I walk or jog, reminding myself to breathe smoothly and rhythmically, and, most important, to relax and release any held tension in my body: "Breathe deeply, belly out on the inhale and in on the exhale. Roll your shoulders back and down, away from your ears. Be loose. Be soft. Smile, don't grimace. Let your arms be free, swinging them from side to side."

I also hold my hands in a *mudra*, or hand yoga position, most often *chin mudra*, which is a well-known and very comforting position where the pads of the thumb and index finger join together. Chin mudra expresses our desire to realize our divinity and become one with cosmic consciousness. (There are twenty-five mudras in Hatha yoga, including sacred body postures, eye positions, breathing techniques, and hand gestures, that are well worth further study.)

This entire process enables me to fully engage my musculoskeletal system and express the full range of motion. No part of my body is static or held taut. I also remind myself to draw my lower spine toward the earth, which automatically draws in the lower abdominals, engaging the core of the body.

Now, visualize your body performing at its best, and how your vigorous walk gives your heart a great workout, increases circulation, releases endorphins, balances hormones, and thoroughly energizes you. This kind of focus and attitude follows your intention and greatly enhances the benefits of a walking session. Even if you're lost in thought—by golly, you've chosen to get lost in thought (an active form of meditation that can help solve problems). The real challenge comes in refraining from thinking when you don't *need* to think. Again, this will follow your intention. Walking meditation clearly shows the Buddhist precept, "All action is preceded by intention." So how about setting this book aside temporarily and lacing up your shoes? Okay now, off you go.

LOVE YOUR YOGA

Today, nary a destination, resort, or hotel spa opens without including a yoga pavilion. And there are plenty of day spas that also include this sacred space for yoga practice. You may have also noticed that yoga showed up in all three types of physical activity discussed earlier in this chapter. The level—meaning the intensity or gentleness of your yoga practice, along with the speed or flow—with which you move through each yoga *asana* (posture) determines the overall benefits of the yoga session. Regardless of which yoga style you choose, you'll enjoy it. I know I do! I love my yoga!

Yoga works on a deep level, and while some of you may already understand the magic I refer to, others might need a brief introduction. So let's devote some special time to understanding this extraordinary practice. Whether or not you live it, you probably at least know of yoga. It has become quite popular in the United States over the past ten years. We Americans, however, in large number tend to focus on the physical aspects of yoga, working through the asanas and regarding the practice primarily in terms of its fitness component. This is valid to a degree. Yoga is one of my primary physical activities, coupled with other regular cardio activities such as running, brisk walking, biking, and swimming. But yoga can go much further, becoming a lifestyle and a profound spiritual practice. There are many yoga styles: Hatha, Integral, Iyengar, Para, Sivananda, Ashtanga, Anusara, Tantra, Kundalini, and Bikram, to name but a few. Also, there are thousands of yoga postures to enjoy. When it comes to yoga philosophy and asanas, you could go a lifetime and never run out of things to learn! Now let's take a quick journey through the history, virtues, and possibilities of yoga.

A Philosophy to Live By

Yoga's been around for over five thousand years. An ancient Hindu practice, literally meaning "union" or "yoke," it represents a philosophy for living life, a way of joyfully transforming our inner and outer worlds. As an elemental part of *Ayurveda* (a sister science to yoga), it's seen as the intertwining of mind, body, spirit, *and* environment into mutually supportive relationships.

What does all this weaving and connecting accomplish? A lot! People who practice yoga regularly are less anxious and less stressed (yoga lowers cortisol levels). These individuals tend to have lower blood pressure and more efficient heart function. Yoga can reduce asthma attacks, as well as the amount of insulin needed by diabetics. There's a correlation between yoga and clearing of the coronary arteries, and yoga postures and breathing techniques can significantly help back injuries, along with arthritis and rheumatism.

Some call their yoga practice "meditation in motion," and indeed it can have a meditative effect by virtue of the concentration you place on your breath and body while performing asanas.

Its ability to simultaneously calm and invigorate distinctly heightens awareness.

Yoga increases the body's flexibility, releases tension, promotes better blood circulation, speeds up metabolism, improves digestion, and enhances endocrine and organ functions. It helps us fully realize our inner and outer beauty. Our minds calm down, our limbs become long and lean, and our mind-body physiology functions from a place of wholeness. We radiate peace, joy, and vibrant energy.

When it comes to asanas, yoga is the most flexible physical activity—pun intended! It's a wonderful activity to perform on its own or with other activities. Alone, it can provide a complete workout, balancing and aligning every part of you, including your spine, muscles, and breath. Depending on the speed and duration of your yoga session, it can be a cardio workout, as in Ashtanga or Bikram yoga. Also, like weight lifting, yoga can strengthen your muscles through resistance exercises, except instead of using barbells and machines, you use your body's own weight.

Pranayama is an integral part of yoga. We connect the mind and body through the breath. Also, yoga is a great prelude to meditation, given how yoga profoundly quiets down the mind and body, allowing us to go deeply into the silence within, where we commune with spirit.

As for the best time to practice yoga, any time is the right time. Personally, I enjoy practicing yoga postures before rolling out of bed in the morning—yes, bed yoga! I also practice a flow of postures (from ten to twenty minutes, depending on the postures I choose to do and their pacing) before hitting the great outdoors for a jog. I also practice in the evening, because it helps release any held tension from the day. Yoga is also the perfect take-along practice on my travels. When I'm alone at night in a hotel room, yoga is a wonderful way to unwind and prepare for deep sleep.

You don't have to do a lengthy practice every day to realize the benefits. Daily practice optimizes yoga's delicious powers of mind-body rejuvenation, yet one, two, or three postures at a time can do the trick. Whether at intervals throughout your workday, at home before you take a walk, or as a warm-up to a cardio workout, doing a few postures provides tremendous benefit. Consistent use of a few basic postures goes a long way toward loosening up physical constraints and opening yourself up to new possibilities of mental and emotional experience. A condensed routine could include a forward bend, a back bend, a twist, and a restorative asana, such as child's pose or corpse pose.

Sacred Energy

In yoga, we teach about the seven *chakras*, or energy centers, located along the spine. The chakras relate to various areas of life experience. The root chakra, at the base of the spine, relates to our base desires or survival needs; the second, or navel chakra, to creativity, sexuality, pleasure, and relationships; the third, also known as the solar plexus, to issues of self-esteem, personal power, and manifesting our desires; the fourth, or heart chakra, to love and compassion; the throat chakra to will and self-expression; the sixth, or third-eye chakra, to intuition, concentration, and wisdom; and the crown chakra, on the top of the head, to our purest potential, divine consciousness, and universal spirituality.

Yoga, on its most basic level, consists of yoga postures, or asanas, that stretch and massage the spine, and calm the nervous system. These postures, when practiced together with breathwork and meditaion, will optimize the flow of electromagnetic energy, or *prana*, through the mind-body physiology and also activate or open the *chakras*, or energy centers, with the ultimate goal being to awaken the *kundalini* energy. Kundalini yoga (recommended under skilled instruction, given its potential for far-reaching and potentially devastating effects), aims to raise "the serpent power," normally coiled and dormant in the lower back, from the psychic centers, into the spinal column, and up to the brain so that fear and creative energies may be sublimated into pure spiritual energy. Here, you can experience true liberation, a triumph that can take a lifetime of practice. This energy is known to trigger extraordinary visionary, auditory, and other sensory experiences.

Ultimately, as your focus travels from the root chakra up toward the crown chakra, vibrational frequency and intensity grows. Balancing the chakras can result in optimal vitality and health, because this energetic system also very much relates to our physicality. Through the chakra network, the mind, body, and spirit are woven together as one holistic system. Imbalances in one's chakra system may show up as a mental or physical dysfunction, or disease.

As spiritual beings, we strive to open all the chakras to their optimal energy flow and vibration, enabling ourselves to become harmonious, open channels to the universal spirit. Bringing a harmonious and balanced self into everything we do becomes our gift to the world and our legacy when we leave this earthly plane.

Many spas integrate chakra-balancing into their services. Meditation, visualization, energy work (such as Reiki), massage, aura balancing, shiatsu, acupuncture, color therapy, and toning (using sound) are all ways to realign the chakra system.

The Asanas (Postures)

Asanas fall into six categories: standing postures, inversions, back bends, forward bends, twists, and meditational (also called "restorative") asanas. This last group is used between more difficult asanas and at the end of each yoga session, but may indeed be used individually at any time. Lie in a restorative posture for at least five minutes, allowing mind and body time to assimilate and fully experience the enhanced energy flow and heightened consciousness generated from practice. Then carry this awareness out into your field of activity.

Breathe! Integral to yoga is remembering to breathe—smoothly and evenly. Our vital energy flows freely through breath. As a general guideline, inhale when extending the body, and exhale when flexing it.

Stay True to Yourself: The golden rule for yoga enthusiasts, especially those attending classes, is to resist the competitive urge. If you find yourself trying to one-up your teacher or the person on the mat beside you, then you've missed the point. Move to your own rhythm and within your own physical limits. Honor your body and allow it to go as far as it wants to go—no farther. It's valuable to play around and inch a bit farther in the asanas but not to the point of pain or injury. Concentrate on *your* body and breath. This deep focus allows your body to fully let go and sink deeper into the asana. And what a delicious release!

Plenty of Resources: Speaking of classes, I encourage you to take one. Or look into the excellent DVDs and cable-TV shows offered. *Lilias! Yoga and You*, hosted by Lilias Folan, is one of my favorite television shows, and can be seen on many PBS stations. She has done yoga on TV since I was a kid, and today she's as beautiful, serene, and limber as ever. Living Arts DVDs are also exceptional in quality. *Yoga Journal*, *Yoga + Joyful Living*, and *ascent* are excellent monthly magazines; and www.iyogalife.com, www.yoga.com, www.yogamates.com, and www.yogasite.com are all great websites.

PLEASURE-HEALING RITUAL: Simply Yoga

We've already enjoyed the profound effect tadasana (mountain pose) can have on us. Now I'd like to share a few more asanas with you. Naturally, every one of you reading this is at a different level of understanding and experience when it comes to yoga; however, these asanas are so easy, everyone can appreciate them. I invite you to become familiar with these simple stretches, all easy to incorporate into your day. Don't let their simplicity fool you though, for each is incredibly rejuvenating.

Do these one at a time or in combination, depending on what part of your body needs TLC. Breathe smoothly and fluidly while performing these asanas, and pay attention to every sensation in your body. Naturally, it's best to develop a regular practice, in whatever way works for you.

The neck and shoulders are particularly vulnerable to stress and tension. These stretches profoundly release stress and built-up tension in these muscles and, when practiced regularly, can prevent chronic neck and shoulder pain. ("Forward head thrust" is quite the problem these days in orthopedics, and yoga can certainly provide tremendous therapy for this problem.) These stretches can also realign the upper spine, allowing for greater blood flow to the brain, which helps promote calm, clear thinking. Do each stretch while breathing naturally and smoothly. Hold it for as long as you desire. Counter with a stretch toward the opposite side, where applicable.

Ear to shoulder: Either standing or seated with feet flat on the floor, spine straight, and head stacked over your shoulders, gently roll your right ear down to your shoulder. Breathe and release any tension you feel through the left side of your neck out into your shoulder. Gently bring your head back upward. Repeat on the other side.

Head side-to-side: Standing or sitting straight, turn your head to the right as far as comfortable. Try to look toward the wall behind you, stretching the muscles and tissues around your neck and also your eyes (eye yoga!). This twists the cervical spine, enhancing side-to-side range of motion, a move we use often. Repeat on the other side.

Shoulder shrugs: Sit or stand up straight. Inhaling, raise your shoulders up to your ears. Now, exhaling, thoroughly release your shoulders downward as far as they'll go. Feel the release of held tension.

Shoulder rolls: With your spine straight, stand with both feet flat on the floor and arms relaxed by your sides. Roll your shoulders in a circular pattern, moving upward and back. Repeat several times, and then go in the opposite direction.

Arm, hand, and shoulder stretch: Standing or seated, with your spine straight, interlace your fingers in front of your heart center. Slowly turn and reach your interlaced hands outward and away from the heart center. Reach your outstretched palms as far as you can, feeling your shoulder blades round out. This is a nice stretch! Feel it in your fingers, palms, wrists, forearms, shoulders, and upper-back area. Breathe smoothly and fluidly. Now slowly raise your outstretched palms toward the sky, following them with your gaze. Feel the extension through your arms and sides as you stretch upward as far as you can. Take several breaths, and then bring your arms back outward from your heart center. Finally, turn your palms inward, drawing them in toward your chest. Release them down by your sides.

Modified *trikonasana* (triangle pose): This posture provides a wonderful lateral stretch through the entire side of the body. With your legs shoulder-width apart, ground the soles of your feet into the earth. Relax your arms by your sides. Keep your torso facing forward throughout this stretch. Now, raise your right arm toward the sky, next to your ear with your palm facing inward. The other arm is by your left side, palm facing in toward your body. Now begin to move your torso toward the left side, reaching as far as comfortable with your outstretched right arm. The other arm glides downward along your left leg, with your hand coming to rest on your leg. Repeat on the other side. Remember to be soft and breathe!

Downward-facing dog: It's so enjoyable to watch my pooch Luna do her downward-facing dog stretch. And she does it often. We humans could definitely learn from this. Downward-facing dog is a wonderful full-body stretch and strenghtener—one of my faves actually! It's an inversion posture that gives your heart a break from gravity. It releases overall tension, increases flexibility (great hamstring stretch!), and lengthens and strengthens the entire spinal column and abdominals; plus, it's quite the energizer. It also lubricates the muscles, joints, tendons, and bones of the hands, arms, shoulders, back, ankles, and more. This posture even stimulates our bones to retain calcium, helping to prevent bone deterioration and loss, and even possibly stimulating bone growth when done regularly. It'll also strengthen and shape muscles you didn't know you had!

(1) Kneel on all fours with your knees under your hip bones and your hands one hand's distance forward from your shoulders and shoulder-width apart. Spread your

fingers open wide, with your hands pressing into the earth or your mat (or towel or carpet) through the base area of your fingers. (2) Firm your inner thighs inward and back, and draw your tailbone toward your heels. Curl your toes into the floor. Exhaling, lift your buttocks toward the sky, pressing into the floor through your hands. If your heels don't reach the floor, that's okay; with practice, they will. (3) Let your head hang between your arms. Keep your buttocks extending upward toward the sky while reaching deeply into the earth through your hands. Breathe smoothly and naturally for several breaths. (4) Release your body back down on all fours. Sit back on your heels while lowering your torso and head down toward the floor into child's pose, a wonderfully restorative posture (covered in detail on the next page).

If you feel pressure in your wrists while doing this asana, roll up a towel and place it under the back heel of your wrists to alleviate excessive pressure.

Seated spinal twist: Twists are wonderful for calming the central nervous system. This stretch is also so rejuvenating for the spine; it turns and lengthens it while enhancing blood flow and flexibility. Spinal twists can also release tension in the intercostal muscles, very deep muscles on either side of the spine. Twists enhance side-to-side range of motion, thereby strengthening and toning the entire spine. Sit up straight, drawing your tailbone downward into your chair. Cross your right leg over your left leg. Now gently place your left hand on your outer-right knee area, all the while breathing smoothly and gently. Lengthen upward. Then, exhaling, twist your torso around to the right, looking over your right shoulder. Hold this position as long as you comfortably can. Inhaling, release and come out of the pose the same way you went in. Repeat on the other side.

Cat and cow pose: This combination stretch is divine for increasing the spine's flexibility. Kneel on all fours, with your knees underneath your hips, and your hands one hand's distance from your shoulders to alleviate wrist tension. Bring your back into a neutral, "table," position, parallel to the floor. Keep your tailbone gently drawn toward your heels. Inhaling, drop your belly toward the mat (or towel or carpet), rounding your back downward as far as it will go (like a cow), and bring your head up and forward, while allowing the sit bones (the bones of the pelvis under the flesh of your buttocks when you're sitting) to blossom outward. Exhaling, round your back toward the sky, like a cat, dropping your head downward between your arms and drawing your pelvis down toward the earth. Repeat this sequence to your breath, or hold each posture for several breaths if you'd like. See your spine as an undulating wave, flowing smoothly and fluidly from cow into cat pose. This is a wonderful vitalizer for the spine.

Child's pose: This resorative posture is tremendously nurturing. Kneel on all fours on your yoga mat (or towel or carpet). Exhaling, sit back on your heels. Release your forehead forward onto the floor or a folded towel. Now bring your arms back along your hips with palms facing up. Settle into this positon. Feel how your thighs compress into your torso. Breathe smoothly and fluidly, releasing even deeper with each breath. Feel how each breath massages all of your internal organs. When you're ready to come out, be sure to draw your tailbone toward your heels and come back up onto all fours on the inhale. Repeat as desired.

Urdhva hastasana (upward salute or arms reaching upward pose): I have my students go directly from tadasana (mountain) into upward salute to further the spine lengthening and aligning benefits.

(1) Begin in tadasana (mountain) pose, covered earlier. (2) Inhaling, sweep your arms out and overhead toward the heavens with your palms facing each other. Feel the expansion through the chest. (3) Spread your fingers open, charge them with energy, and stretch them toward the sky. (4) Gently gaze upward, giving yourself a slight back bend if you'd like. Keep your tailbone gently drawn downward toward the earth. Feel the magnificant stretch throughout your entire body. (5) Exhaling, release your arms downward into prayer pose, with your palms together in front of your heart center. Take a breath or two here, contemplating your own heart as the center of love and compassion, and then release your arms back down to your sides.

Modified uttanasana (**forward bend**): This posture is profound in its ability to release lower-back tension. However, if you have issues with your lower back, proceed with caution. Only move as far as your body wants to go, and if it feels tight or inflexible, bend your knees slightly when performing this asana.

(1) Stand in tadasana (mountain pose) with your arms loose by your sides. (2) Gently float your chin toward your chest. Let your head fully release. Feel the wonderful stretch along the back of your neck and shoulders. (3) Now begin to roll your body downward. Let your arms and head dangle down and forward, with your body following. I like to imagine the spinal column as a string of pearls. Imagine floating downward toward the earth, pearl by pearl, vertebra by vertebra. (4) When you are as low as you can go, take several breaths, and then slowly unfurl back up into tadasana. Remember to keep your tailbone drawn toward the earth throughout.

Viparita karani (**legs-up-the-wall pose**): Legs-up-the-wall, shoulder stand, head stand, forward bend, and downward-facing dog are all inverted poses. It's believed that inverting our bodies redirects the flow of prana (the life-force energy) inward toward the vital organs. It increases blood circulation to the brain, face, neck, and thorax and improves functioning of the adrenal, pituitary, and thyroid glands, as well as pelvic circulation. Try inverting your body every day, and relish in this posture's energizing, rejuvenating, and balancing effects.

(1) Sit on the floor with one shoulder and hip next to the wall and your knees bent. Turn your legs upward along the wall, perpendicular to the ground, lying on your back. At first, you may not be able to place your buttocks flush against the wall. As you release and gain more flexibility, you'll be able to bring them closer. Another option is to have a folded blanket or pillow close by to place under your buttocks and sacrum area, elevating your torso a bit higher. This further inverts your heart against the flow of gravity, reversing vascular flow and feeding freshly oxygenated blood to your brain. (2) Bring your arms out by your sides, or form them into a soft U shape, with your hands facing above your head. Draw your shoulders down away from your ears. (3) Lengthen your neck along the floor, making sure your chin is lower than your forehead (place a folded towel under your head, if desired). (4) Check in with your body and make sure there are no areas that feel strained. (5) Breathe smoothly and evenly as long as you desire. (6) To come out of the pose, bend your knees to your chest and release them to the side and onto the floor. Plant your hands onto the floor to raise your body.

Virabhadrasana II (warrior II): This powerful standing pose provides numerous benefits, such as increased stamina and improved strength in the hips, legs, and ankles. It's important to perform it correctly. If you're uncertain, seek out yoga instruction (whether through an instructor, a website, or DVD) to assist you with the proper technique. This posture is specifically helpful for releasing tension in the hip-flexor area, where the powerful psoas muscle is located. Restriction in the hips, and specifically, tight psoas, can cause a ripple effect through the body, resulting in lower-back pain, tight hamstrings, and more. Try to open up your hips in some way each and every day. This posture gives you a good start. To find your center (the place where your energy is distributed evenly) in virabhadrasana II, start by grounding yourself in tadasana (mountain pose). When you feel your mind settle within the relaxed steadiness of tadasana, then prepare to begin virabhadrasana II.

(1) Step your feet apart three and a half to four feet. Plant your feet into the earth like roots, connecting through all corners of your feet. Raise both your arms parallel to the floor, with palms facing downward. (2) Keep your tailbone drawn downward. Pivot your right foot inward to a forty-five-degree angle, while pivoting your left foot ninety degrees to the left. Turn your head to the left and bend at your left knee. Keep the right hip opened toward the back. Breathe smoothly and fluidly. You can stay in this position as long as you desire. Repeat in the opposite direction.

Shavasana (corpse pose): Often used to begin or end a yoga session, this relaxation or restorative pose allows your mind-body physiology to sink deeply into the earth, which can be seen as a death-like experience, hence its name. Corpse pose helps us to see that the bodies we inhabit are not the true essence of our being, and encourages us to embrace our "witness" self, alleviating the intense fear and anxiety associated with death. This increased self-awareness of our true nature helps us to remain detached and calm amid the stress of our daily lives. On a restorative level, all of our major muscles, tendons, joints, and organs release, allowing for the ultimate in de-stressing, liberation, and peace.

(1) Make sure you are warm and comfortable. Have a blanket handy if need be, and a rolled-up blanket or bolster to place under your knees if your lower back is tight. Lying on your back, spread your arms and legs out comfortably from your body. Your palms are upward, and your feet are left to fall naturally outward. Tilt your head back slightly so that it rests comfortably. (2) Close your eyes and let your breath deepen. Let your body become soft and heavy as it relaxes into the earth. As you relax, feel your entire body rising and falling with each breath. (3) Scan your body from your toes upward to the crown of your head, looking for any tension or constriction. Consciously relax and release any tense areas you find. Rock or wiggle them if need be to release even further. (4) Release all control of your mind, body, and breath. Let your body move deeper and deeper into a profound state of relaxation. (5) Stay in shavasana for at least five minutes; the longer, the better for assimilating its sublime benefits. (6) To release, deepen your breath, wiggle your fingers and toes, and then stretch your arms overhead. Energize your fingers and toes, and reach as far as you can in opposing directions for a pow-

erful full-body stretch. Draw your knees in toward your chest and roll over onto your side into a fetal position. When you're ready, use your hands on the floor to lift your body up into a seated position. (This would be an excellent time to go into meditation, as you've profoundly calmed down the mind-body physiology.) Ahh! Take this consciousness into your interaction with the world.

Through your practice, remember to breathe and honor your body. I recommend practicing these asanas in bare feet, but if you practice at work, stocking feet or flat shoes are fine, depending on whether you're doing "mat" work on the floor, or seated postures. Remember, don't go any farther than your body wants to go!

EVERYBODY DANCE

Dance resonates deeply in us and comes so naturally. Look at babies; the moment they make it up on their feet, they're dancing! They don't know they're dancing, but the way they let their limbs move freely about is a most primal form of dance. I love watching and being inspired by this!

Dance makes us feel powerful, and when we feel powerful, we feel good. Dancing gives the heart a great workout, increases the flow of oxygenated blood through the body, and starts those endorphins flowing, thoroughly energizing us. And when we dance, we let go. We unknot, unfurl, and disengage our brains, letting the body take over.

Because of the therapeutic aspects of dance, there are even dance-therapy organizations where expressive movement is used as a healing tool for personal expression and psychological or emotional wellness. Dance therapists work with clients with physical disabilities, addiction issues, sexual-abuse histories, eating disorders, and other concerns.

You may know the more traditional and contemporary types of dance (*Dancing with the Stars* and *So You Think You Can Dance* have awakened this consciousness for many), such as the waltz, the fox-trot, polka, rumba, ballet, and funky jazz, but how about some alternative dance forms? I've occasionally attended an ecstatic, or trance, dance, which is a most primordial way to move the body, free the mind, and connect with spirit. Shamans and indigenous peoples have practiced trance dance for thousands of years. This ancient transformative and healing technique is becoming quite popular.

Anyone can dance. Just like the Sufi whirling dervishes, you swirl, chant, and channel as you dance your way to ecstasy. Turn on your favorite music, close your eyes, and let spirit move you. I dare you!

PLEASURE-HEALING RITUAL: Move Your Soul with Ecstatic Dance

One of my favorite total-awareness workouts is ecstatic dance, or trance dance. Trust the process and let it unfold organically. You may experience yourself as spaceless and timeless. Not a great deal of space is required because the dance largely happens within, but having more space allows you to make more expansive movements and get the juices flowing more quickly. It's all good.

1. Turn on your musical selection, one that allows you to tune in to the rhythm and move freely. Begin by standing with your feet parallel to your shoulders, and let your body and mind relax.

2. Close your eyes if you're comfortable in your surroundings so that your eyes will "see" the vast inner landscape of your consciousness.

3. Become aware of your breathing, inhaling and exhaling deeply, thoroughly filling your lungs. Doing this for a few minutes awakens the energizer, the experiencer within.

4. Relax and allow your body to move to the rhythm. Soon you'll feel prana (life-force energy) moving through your body. At this point, the dancer disappears, and you become the dance. You've awakened spirit. You may experience profound emotions, a sense of letting go, and a peaceful connection to your immortal self.

This process can go on for thirty minutes or so. When I'm sweating—"sweating my prayers," as Gabrielle Roth, the goddess of the dance and founder of the popular 5Rhythms method is known to say—I know I've arrived. It's pure ecstasy. When the music ends, take several minutes to be still and integrate your experience.

MEDITATION IN MOTION

Whatever activity you're involved in, the more you relax while moving, the more positive the experience *and* the more efficiently you build muscle and burn fat. When you're tense, you tighten muscles that should stay slack, and your movements become wooden, tiring you faster. Breath awareness and use of a mantra are simple ways to help relax and be present during physical activity. Silently repeat a favorite word, use ujjayi breath (see chapter 3), and focus intently on your bodily movements and posture. Your workout will benefit tremendously from these extra measures. Naturally, movement activities such as yoga and tai chi are very much about the mind-body connection and being present during practice, but we can bring this awareness into all of our physical-fitness activities.

Our bodies are an incredible gift, endowed with limitless potential. As the great, ancient yogi sage Saraha said, "Here in the body are the sacred rivers: here are the sun and the moon, as well as all the pilgrimage places. I have not encountered another temple as blissful as my own body." Honor the sacredness of your body *and* your mind; become a true physical activist. Imbue every moment possible with glorious, playful, vitalizing movement.

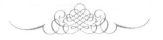

CHAPTER 7

TOUCH ME, FEEL ME

Remember only the beautiful things that you have felt and seen and experienced. If your five senses behold only the good, then your mind will be a garden of blossoming soul qualities.

—PARAMAHANSA YOGANANDA

"I was so touched by what you said." "We've lost touch with each other." Truly, touch serves as a metaphor for a deep and soulful connection with others. As sensuality practices go, touch is such a primal need, and one of our most intimate and powerful forms of communication. When you're "in touch," you're energetically connecting with another sentient being, human or otherwise. When you practice self-care and care for others, you take delight in maintaining connections and in the shared pleasure (and healing) of being in touch. And there are so many ways to show this caring, whether over distance or in person, on the level of the psyche, or on the physical level. If you listen to your heart, you'll know when compassion calls upon you to send loving-kindness to another, whether by sending positive energy, praying, picking up the phone, dropping a quick note, wrapping your arms around a grieving neighbor, or embracing a loved one for the pure joy of it.

Everyone has his or her own sensuality quotient and style of touch. Consider how you might escalate the element of touch in your relationships while honoring appropriate boundaries. See this as a practice. Touch your friend's arm as she tells you a heartfelt story, hug your teenager, massage the neck and shoulders of a special senior in your life, or walk arm in arm with your significant other. Touching is a form of communicating, and the benefits go beyond physical health. If you touch others with sensitivity, you relate to them with sensitivity.

Regardless of cultural background, our sensuality and ability to be intimate with others forms early on. Every family has informal rules about touch and verbal communication, and this often-unconscious orientation can be deeply ingrained, staying with us throughout our lifetime. We can embrace this orientation, allowing it to make us who we are. But many of us may find that embarking on our own sensory journey, where we slowly and assuredly nourish and delight body, mind, and soul, allows us to deepen our intimacy with ourselves, our loved ones, our community, and our environment.

SEXUAL HEALING

In exploring touch, I'd be remiss if I didn't include a brief exploration of sexual intimacy and healing. Many high-profile spas today offer seminars and workshops on sacred loving. Healing traditions from earliest times to the present include nurturing of creative and sexual energies as a sacred expression of the divine. Divine energy flows through all things, creating and giving life. When we tap into this energy, we become more loving, beyond the traditional meaning of sexual intimacy. Compassion, enchantment, sensuality, commitment, joy, and many other emotions come into play. Naturally, an important facet of love *is* our sexuality and how we express it. Blockages in sexual energy impede our otherwise freeflowing ability to express ourselves and realize our desires. If you seek to vitalize your creative or sexual energy, it's a valuable practice to look inward, reflecting on who you are, why you're here, and what would make you truly happy. Clearly see your desires, visualize them, and give them a voice. If you haven't a clue what would make you happy, how can you share it or seek it out? And, yes, this includes self-love, the ultimate form of sacred touch. Positively affirm your desired outcome through introspection and questioning.

Perhaps you've heard the common expression, "Sexuality begins in the mind, not the genitals." However, a number of saboteurs (stressors) can take us away from our most loving, libidinous self. Feeling the love takes a desire and commitment on our part. It's very easy in today's stressful and time-starved world to let sexual satisfaction fall by the wayside. Some of you may want to renew this wonderful relationship with your sexual self.

The Tantric Approach

In *tantra* yoga, pursuit of sexual pleasure has long been a form of sacrament, considered as essential to nurturing life as food and water. The ultimate manual on tantra lovemaking, the Kama Sutra, was written by Vatsyayana two thousand years ago, about the same time as the Bible's book of Revelation. Tantra is a mélange of worship, ritual, meditation, and mysticism. In Tantrism, sexual pleasure isn't seen as the priority, although that doesn't mean the experience isn't fulfilling; it's quite the opposite. This tradition teaches that knowledge leads to direct experience of God, where you and your partner's bodies meet the spiritual elements within and around you. To the yogi, tantric worship transforms orgiastic energy into a spiritual force that drives the worshipper to the divine. Lovers merge through their breath and consciousness. In other words, the true pleasure of sex doesn't come from orgasm but rather in receiving and satisfying your partner.

Whereas classical yoga seeks to overcome the distractions of the senses through detachment, tantra not only accepts them but also assigns them a central role in the quest for holy enlightenment. In tantra, all the senses are engaged; no experience is avoided. Silken robes; body paint; sensuous fabrics; candles; oils; fragrant flowers; lavish cushions; and edibles, such as fruits, champagne, and chocolates, are kept close at hand to titillate the tongue and refresh the senses. I encourage further study of the Kama Sutra.

In its original Sanskrit, the text outlines a comprehensive prescription for pleasurable living, and incorporates aspects of mythology and astrology at length. And, of course, there are the sixty-four enlightening "art of sex" passages. A big reason for the Kama Sutra's lasting fame and centuries of devoted practitioners is that it equally emphasizes our spiritual desires and sexual satisfaction, taking into consideration our human need to feel appreciated and emotionally connected, which is part of sacred touch!

SO TOUCHED!

We experience so much through the skin we're in. Our skin, the body's largest organ, includes as many as five million touch receptors with three thousand in a single fingertip. These touch receptors send messages along the spinal cord to the brain. A simple touch with loving intent can reduce the heart rate and lower blood pressure. Touch also stimulates the brain to produce endorphins, the body's natural pain suppressors and mood enhancers. Maybe this is why a mother's hug can make almost anything better. On a physical level, touch is a powerful healer, eliciting physiological changes that nurture and calm. It's true! Muscles relax, stress diminishes, and a profound sense of calm comes over the person being touched. So reach out and touch someone today, whether yourself or a loved one, and give a hand and arm massage, a neck and shoulder rub, or a full-out hug. It's free, naturally sweet yet nonfattening, good for you, and feels amazing. It's also invigorating; after all, haven't you felt energized after a good hug? Hugs come in endless supplies, so give them out freely.

Massage Therapy

An integral part of touch is massage. Do you know what sustained touch through massage therapy can do? This is not a rhetorical question! As a certified massage therapist, I know well what massage therapy is capable of accomplishing. I try to see my own massage therapist twice a month. She helps me feel whole, coaxing out those holding patterns that get bound up inside my muscles. Besides just plain feeling good (those endorphins!), massage relaxes me, reduces my stress, improves my blood circulation, increases my flexibility, enhances my range of motion, and raises my energy levels.

How does this happen? When your skin is stroked, a pharmacy of natural feel-good chemicals releases into your bloodstream, including natural growth hormones, antidepressants, tranquilizers, and pain relievers, along with immunomodulators and vasodilators. Along with the pain-reducing, blood-pressure-lowering benefits, massage dramatically increases lymph flow, moves toxins out of the system (because skin is a primary pathway for detoxification), and powerfully boosts the immune system.

What else can massage do, you ask? It lowers levels of the "stress hormones" cortisol, norepinephrine, and epinephrine that wreak havoc on the body when uncontrolled. Some types of massage may release old injuries held in a muscle's memory, allowing healing to proceed. Massage stimulates the vagus, one of twelve cranial nerves that influence a variety of bodily functions. One branch of the vagus travels to the gastrointestinal tract, where it facilitates release of food-absorption hormones such as insulin and glucose, making food absorption more efficient.

Stroking or massaging the skin undoubtedly provides numerous rejuvenating and healing benefits for our mind-body health. Bring this into your consciousness, and if you've never experienced the full joy of touch, make an appointment for a massage-therapy treatment, the primary and most popular treatment requested at spas. You can also contact the American Massage Therapy Association to use their locator service and receive qualified recommendations (www.amtamassage.org).

A Style for Every Type

There are many types of massage therapy, along with a variety of beneficial results. Traditional Swedish massage involves manipulation of the muscles and tissues. Oriental healing arts, such as shiatsu, concentrate on pressure points and the body's energy flow. Reflexology is a foot or hand massage technique based on the centuries-old Chinese theory that areas of the hands and feet correspond directly to other body parts; namely, organs, glands, and joints. Through gentle pressure and manipulation, tension and blockages are released. Other therapies include aromatherapy, Ayurveda, craniosacral therapy, deep tissue massage, sports massage, Esalen, lymphatic massage, myofascial release, Thai massage, trigger-point therapy (myotherapy), and Watsu (in-water massage, which is heavenly), to name only a few.

Massage professionals may use a combination of techniques, adjusting to customize therapies to your mind-body energy type.

For example, given my muscularity, my therapist uses deep neuro-muscular massage coupled with trigger-point therapy (which eases muscle soreness or contraction by direct finger pressure), which is ideal for my needs. You may want less pressure and more calming strokes, given your level of comfort and need.

With such a variety of massage knowledge and expertise out there, my aim is to ignite your interest to seek out more information on your own, for which the Internet can be beneficial, and numerous courses, videos, and books are also available. In the meantime, realize that massage can bring into your life tremendous healing and relaxation benefits that are very blissful indeed!

Self-Massage

In giving yourself the love and attention you deserve (because you're lovable; give yourself a positive affirmation here!), don't forget to give yourself a daily massage, one of the most organic healing practices for your self-care. Self-massage is a great way to wake up or bed down, because it has a very stabilizing effect while also enhancing alertness and preparing you to better face each day.

The following self-massage technique is incredibly healing and detoxifying. Enjoy it in the morning, coupled with yoga and meditation, to help put everything into glorious perspective. Adjust the amount of pressure you apply to your body according to your comfort level. Some prefer a light touch, some prefer firm pressure, and still others want a more vigorous massage for its stimulating qualities. Do what feels most natural and pleasant to you. Also, be aware of the power of your hands and the energy they transfer. Bringing this awareness to massaging yourself and others greatly enhances the overall experience. To grasp this point, try closing your eyes, breathing deeply, and "listening" to the tissues and bones beneath your hands as you massage yourself or a loved one. Envision the body with a sense of wholeness and interconnectedness rather than seeing it as having separate parts. Intuitively performing a massage with this intent and in this manner enhances the quality of the experience.

To prepare, begin by mixing a bit of organic plant oil (the "carrier" oil) with your favorite aromatic essential oil. Select the essential or plant oil for its calming, cooling, or stimulating properties, whatever you need at the moment (see the next chapter for more on aromatherapy). It's best to use organic plant oils labeled "pure cold" or "expeller pressed" as the carrier oil to add your essential oils into, ensuring that chemicals won't be applied to and absorbed through your skin. Sesame oil is a good all-around selection for a carrier oil because of its absorbability and potent antioxidant qualities. For dry skin, try sweet-almond, rice-bran, and avocado oils or ghee (clarified butter). For oily skin, you might choose sweet-almond, canola, grapeseed, kukui, mustard, or safflower oil, using only a minimal amount on oilier skin. For sensitive skin, use cooling oils, such as sweet-almond, coconut, olive, and sunflower oil. Any of these oils balance normal skin. Don't use mineral oil, because it's drying and doesn't penetrate the skin.

PLEASURE-HEALING RITUAL: Self-Massage

Following is the Ayurvedic self-massage approach, called *abhyanga*. Be sure to give yourself the gift of time, at least five minutes but preferably ten, so you can mindfully move through a total body rubdown:

1. Stand or sit on a large bath towel. The towel catches any oil drips.

2. Begin massaging your head for about a minute. Pour a small amount of oil into your palms, working it evenly onto your fingertips and palms. Begin at the top-front hairline area and, using the pads of your fingertips, massage in small, circular motions. Work back to the crown area. Move your scalp with your fingertips to render it more flexible. Work from your temples back to your lower-crown area. Finally, work in small, circular strokes from behind your ears to the center nape. Use more oil as needed.

3. Next, move to your face. With a small amount of oil, work over your face, using upward and outward movements. Gently work around the eyes, outward along the top-brow area and inward along the area underneath. Use a light patting motion under your eyes; no tugging or rubbing! Gently knead around your outer-ear-lobe area, and stroke behind your ears. Use upward strokes on the front of your neck, and up and down strokes on the back of your neck.

4. Stroke back and forth over the area between your neck and shoulders. Use circular motions over your shoulders. With your palm and fingers, stroke back and forth over the top of your arm and forearm, switching to circular strokes over your elbows and wrists. Massage each finger, and then stroke upward on the back of your hand toward your wrist. Massage in a circular, clockwise fashion through your palm area.

5. Use the heel of your hand to stroke up and down over your breastbone (thorax) area. Use gentle, circular, clockwise strokes over your chest, heart, and abdomen.

6. Reaching behind to your lower back and buttocks, massage in a circular motion. Going as far up as possible, stroke back and forth vertically on your back.

7. Use long, back and forth vertical strokes on your upper leg (front and back); smaller, circular strokes at your knee; and long, back and forth strokes on your lower leg. Continue to your ankles.

8. Use upward strokes along the tops of your feet. Then gently massage each toe. Briskly stroke back and forth along your soles.

Make self-massage part of your meditative practice, in the sense of communing with self. Be fully present with yourself when performing this amazing ritual. Set the intention of sending loving energy to yourself. Breathe smoothly, deeply, and evenly as you massage. Let go of any distractions that arise. Any tension that you feel will melt away as you luxuriate in this mood-enhancing practice. This entire process allows your mind to profoundly settle down. If possible, relax for a few minutes after your massage and before bathing. Use a gentle body wash and tepid water to shower or bathe.

At the very least, massage your scalp, hands, and feet at any point during the day or before going to bed. These are rich energy centers, with an extensive network of nerves for inducing deep relaxation. I particularly enjoy massaging my feet with an organic lotion and then covering them with organic cotton socks before bedtime. You'll experience sound slumber and maybe even a sweet dream or two!

Use self-massage wherever and whenever the yearning arises. Do you have sore muscles or inflamed tendons? Spend a few moments massaging them. Do your feet hurt? Kick off your shoes and spend a few minutes with your tootsies. Got an upset tummy? Gently massage your stomach in a clockwise direction, which helps digestion and tones this area. Are you a little too jazzed to go to sleep? Treat yourself to a hand, foot, or scalp massage; then crawl into bed and enjoy deep, blissful sleep, not to mention moisturized skin and scalp.

I hope this information on touch has touched your world and that you'll regard your loving touch as the holistic and healing ritual that it is.

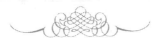

CHAPTER 8

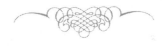

HEAVEN SCENT

Smell is a potent wizard that transports us across thousands of miles and all the years we have lived.

—HELEN KELLER

Freshly mown grass, baby powder, a bouquet of roses, a fragrant pinot noir, chocolate, freshly ground coffee, the air after a thunderstorm, or my husband's shirt—all offer evocative scents for me. I'm sure you can think of a few of your own. Reflect on some of your favorite aromas, the memories they conjure, and how they make you feel. Yes, fragrance has the power to stir something deep within us—and with good reason!

THE POWER OF SCENT

Biologically, smell and memory are linked. The olfactory nerve is only one of a dozen cranial nerves that lead directly to the brain. The olfactory membrane in our nasal passages has millions of scent receptor cells. When aroma molecules bind with these receptors, electrical impulses go to the brain's smell center, signaling the cerebral cortex to send information to the limbic system, the seat of our emotions, memories, intuition, and sexual response. The limbic system also influences hormone levels and the immune system, and interacts with the neocortex area of the brain, the center of higher mental functioning, hence the connection between our sense of smell and our thoughts, behaviors, emotions, desires, and moods. The brain has the ability to process and recall over ten thousand different scents, which explains why every aromatic encounter we have communicates messages to the brain, evoking memories that have a far-reaching effect on our consciousness.

Also, as mentioned earlier, our sense of smell enhances digestion. Smelling your food before taking that first bite starts the digestive process by getting saliva to flow in your mouth. Savoring the smell of our food brings us more enjoyment from our meal. So inhale through your nose before putting that bite of food into your mouth. Sensual people make a habit of savoring the smell *and* taste of their food. At your next meal or snack, spend several moments smelling your food before consuming it. Allow the rich smell of that spaghetti Bolognese to fill your nose. Enjoy the yeasty smell of that Italian bread. Let the scent of freshly squeezed citrus juice uplift you.

MINDFULNESS THROUGH SCENT

Given our emphasis on a mindfulness approach to pleasure healing, consider that the aromas of lavender, rose, apple, and a variety of other flowery or fruity fragrances elicit relaxation and reduce anxiety. As we relax, we're better able to practice mindfulness—and also ease into deep meditation. Each of us will have our own special scents that elicit relaxation and feelings of well-being, and they're usually ones that have strong emotional connections for us, often from childhood, such as Mom's freshly baked apple pie or the fresh smell of line-dried bedsheets. The key is to find those special aromas that elicit relaxation for you. And when you find these special aromas, you'll know you can rely upon them again and again to bring on deep feelings of serenity.

Placing your favorite scent (especially essential oils) on your pulse points (such as your temples or wrists) or in your environment will allow you to slip into meditation with ease every time. If meditation is a challenge for you, train your nervous system to associate these aromas with your meditation time by introducing some form of calming aroma, or even sound (see chapter 9), into your environment. Over time, you'll be able to evoke a deep meditative state by simply thinking about the aroma.

Keep It Fresh

There are definitely toxic smells in our environment. Consider your environment at home and work, including outdoor-air quality, outgassing from volatile organic compounds (VOCs), chemicals from personal-care and household-cleaning products, cigarette smoke, traffic congestion, and other factors. You can see why the importance of fresh air is paramount.

Getting fresh air doesn't simply mean standing in your backyard taking deep breaths; it goes deeper than this. Pollutants strip the air of its natural healing components, specifically the *negative ion*. Negative-ion environments are found at the ocean's edge, in pine forests, by waterfalls, and generally anywhere just after a lightning storm. They're also created by the sun's ultraviolet radiation. Negative-ion environments calm you while creating a feeling of exhilaration. When negative-ion environments are disrupted by pollution, the result is *positive ionization*, which can make you feel fatigued, depressed, tense, and irritable, as well as produce negative physical effects, including frequent headaches, allergies, and even asthmatic conditions.

To make sure you get enough fresh air:

- Consider an air cleaner, or filter, for your home and work environments. (I have a medical-grade HEPA air filter in my home.)

- Make sure you can open your windows to circulate fresh air when necessary.

- Surround yourself with green plants, placing the indoor variety around you and making sure you get outdoors among lush foliage. This allows you to take in the prana-rich (life-force infused) air that these plants release. Plants scrub the air of toxins.

- Spend time near a waterfall. In a pinch, take a shower. Both create negative ions.

AROMATHERAPY

For me, taking deep whiffs of my freshly ground cup of coffee in the morning is a special form of aromatherapy, as is planting my nose in my lilac bush out back. However, in the world of the healing arts, aromatherapy has a special meaning. Many ancient cultures used plant aromatics as incense, salves, unguents, natural perfumes, and distilled waters for health purposes. *Aromatherapy* is the art and science of using essential oils (the volatile oils distilled from a variety of plants or plant parts) or hydrosols (also called "floral water," the water remaining after producing essential oils through steam or water distillation) to relax, balance, and stimulate the body, mind, and spirit. As essential oils go, these aromatic concentrates are usually steam distilled from a variety of flowers, roots, leaves, wood, bark, fruit, berries, seeds, and resins or cold pressed from citrus-fruit rinds. Every essential oil has its own distinct aroma, stimulating an array of emotional, psychological, and physical responses. Oils are massaged into the skin in diluted form, inhaled, or placed in baths. With inhalation, essential oils work by releasing a gaseous vapor into the air. The vaporized molecules are absorbed into the bloodstream through the olfactory receptors in the nostrils and through the lungs. When applied externally during massage, in a bath (or hydrotherapy), and in skin-care and simple first-aid products, essential oils not only work their wonders on the skin's multiple layers but also are absorbed through the skin and carried by the bloodstream to muscle tissues, joints, and organs. Aromatherapy is often used in conjunction with skin, hair, and nail treatments; massage therapy; acupuncture; reflexology; herbology; chiropractic; and other holistic treatments.

More doctors, dentists, psychologists, and nurses are using aromatherapy in medical settings, such as hospitals, hospices, and nursing homes. Why all the attention to aromatherapy? Because this truly delightful art and science based on aroma can alleviate stress, calm the fight-or-flight response, promote alertness, induce sleep, lower blood pressure, increase blood circulation, boost the immune system, increase the appetite, and so much more.

Therapeutic Benefits

Essential oils can effect great internal and external healing, whether through inhalation or application to the skin. They can soothe aching muscles and cramps, improve the skin's appearance and function, reduce lung and sinus congestion, enhance metabolic and other bodily functions, and purify our environment. They can treat infections, bruises, minor cuts and abrasions, arthritis, and headaches. Also, aromas can boost confidence, stimulate and motivate, accelerate learning, quell anxiety, dispel anger, engender love, and enhance sexual desire, as well as moisturize; tone; and provide astringency for the skin, hair, and nails; the list goes on and on. Aromas have expansive healing powers, affecting us physically, mentally, emotionally, and spiritually.

But take heed: "aromatherapy" has become a catchphrase for many products, from personal-care products to accessories for the home, such as candles, pillows, and so on. While I fully applaud the attention to this healing therapy, many of these products do not contain pure essential oils. They're diluted and don't reflect what 100-percent-pure essential oils can accomplish. In fact, many of them contain artificial fragrances, a primary cause of allergic reactions. High-quality essential oils are unadulterated and have no synthetic fillers, suspenders, or added mineral oil. Read the label of any aromatherapy product before purchasing, looking for 100-percent-pure essential oils, preferably certified organic.

Everyone has a highly individual reaction to aromas. Here are a few general guidelines for using aromas to care for yourself, balance your emotions, and create a relaxing and revitalizing environment:

Emotional, excitable, or anxious? Use calming oils that are floral, fruity, warm, or sweet: rose, lavender, geranium, orange, lemon balm, basil, clove, or vanilla. They may also relieve restlessness, anxiety, cramps, backache, heart palpitations, or insomnia.

Fiery, jealous, or overly intense? Soothe, clarify, and ease your mind with cooling, sweet, bitter, or astringent oils: sandalwood, mint, rose, jasmine, chamomile, lily, iris, or honeysuckle. These may relieve inflamed emotions like anger, irritability, impatience, or jealousy, as well as ulcers, inflammatory bowel disease, or inflammatory skin conditions.

Sluggish, susceptible to depression, or complacent? Lighten up and enliven with pungent, spicy, stimulating oils: rosemary, lemongrass, eucalyptus, cedar, sage, musk, juniper, clove, marjoram, or peppermint. All of these have energizing qualities that may increase motivation, and release attachment to and retention of food, fluid, fat, relationships, or unhealthy emotions.

PLEASURE-HEALING RITUAL: Aromatherapy

Consider using simple aromatic practices to experience the pleasure-healing aspects of aromatherapy. Whether done at home or work, begin with a few favorites and then expand your repertoire of essential oil usage as you become more comfortable. I've also included incense and smudging rituals here for your consideration. Although not traditional aromatherapy, they serve their healing purpose:

- Mix six to eight (or your preferred amount) drops of your favorite essential oil into one ounce of organic plant oil, and massage your entire body or any area that needs your loving attention. Be fully present during this process, sending yourself loving energy. (Peppermint oil is great for a belly rub! It helps the digestion and calms an upset stomach.)

- Mist your environment. You can do this by mixing a few drops of essential oil and a teaspoon of alcohol with purified water in an atomizer (shake before each use), or use a hydrosol spray (also called "floral water"). You can also mist your sheets and linens, use as a light cologne or body spray, and even use in finger bowls to add a thoughtful and distinctive touch to a special dinner.

- Create your own natural perfume. Add twenty-five drops of any combination of essential oils to one ounce of perfume alcohol, denatured alcohol, or grain alcohol. Create perfume oil by adding to a carrier oil, such as sweet-almond oil.

- Mix five to six drops of essential oil with a quarter cup of water and add to the washing machine's rinse cycle. This won't stain and will have antimicrobial properties, and a hint of the wonderful aroma will remain. Put a few drops of an essential oil such as rosemary on a small piece of fabric, terry cloth, or washcloth and toss in with your dryer load. This is a natural approach to scenting and softening clothes.

- Use a vaporizer or diffuser to float oils into your environment. Peppermint, eucalyptus, and juniper in the bedroom at night help a stuffy head; lavender in the evening calms the overactive mind or jittery nerves; and citrus oils get you going in the morning as well as brighten your mood. Great sleep inducers include chamomile, lavender, marjoram, and neroli. Put a few drops on a tissue or cotton pad, and tuck into your pillow. Similarly, you can scent your space by adding your essential oil to a pan on the stove and simmering to release the aroma into the air.

- Take a steam. For skin conditions or respiratory problems, bring a pan of water just to a boil on the stove, and then move it to a trivet on a stable surface. Add from eight to twelve drops of essential oil. Sit next to this with your head placed comfortably over the pan, and tent a towel over you to create a steam bath. Now take deep, healing breaths.

- Place a small clay diffuser with essential oils in your automobile. This can produce a positive and calming effect, especially when you're caught in traffic.

- Place a drop or two of essential oil on a cool lightbulb. Turn the light on, and the bulb heats the fragrance and disperses it throughout the room. I like to do this when traveling to purify and make the hotel-room air more pleasant. You can also purchase ceramic-diffuser scent rings specifically made for placing on the lightbulb.

- Add essential oils to your personal-care products to enhance their benefits and features. I like adding a few drops of rosemary essential oil to my hair conditioner and a drop of geranium to my facial moisturizer to accentuate a healthy glow. Or purchase items that already contain 100-percent-pure essential oils (preferably certified organic).

- Take a bath with essential oils. Add six to eight drops of your desired essential oils into a small amount of organic plant oil. Fill the tub and add your oil mixture.

Put in the oil toward the end, when the tub is almost full, to experience the oil's full potency.

- Make your own smelling salts by placing one tablespoon of rock salt and ten drops of basil, peppermint, or rosemary essential oil (or a mixture of these) in a small container with a tightly fitting lid. Inhale as desired, stimulating present-moment awareness, clear thought, and an instant pick-me-up.

- Put a few drops of purifying oils on a cotton ball and place it in a plastic bag in your purse when flying to counter the toxic air inside the airplane cabin. Take it out at intervals during your flight and open it up to take several deep breaths into your lungs. Eucalyptus, rosemary, cedarwood, pine, and tea tree are all great antibacterial, antimicrobial oils for this usage.

- Aromatherapy candles are wonderful for meditation, relaxation, and special occasions. Make sure the candle is made with pure essential oils, natural beeswax, or organic soy, and has a natural, lead-free wick.

- *Nag champa* (fragrance from India that derives from the *champa* flower and has a high sandalwood content) incense is one of my favorites for yoga practice. Whatever your incense selection, make certain to indulge in the highest quality possible.

- The Native American practice of *smudging* is a sacred ritual in which loose or bundled aromatic herbs (sage, cedar, copal, yerba santa, and juniper, to name a few) are burned to draw in blessings and purification, and smoke out negative energies. The herbs are lit over a ceramic bowl or smudge pot, and the embers are gently blown to create smoke. Walk through the environment while smudging it. You can use the smoke to purify your body, home, or workplace; or any gathering, healing, or meditation space.

Choosing Essential Oils

While aromatherapy involves any scent that triggers welcome emotions, it's a good idea to begin by selecting an essential oil known to encourage a specific positive response. To best understand and use essential oils, visit your local full-service spa, health-food store, whole-foods market, or, in many instances, yoga studio. My supplier has small bowls of whole coffee beans available to clear the nose "palate" in between smelling the different aromas. Go through the samplers to discover how the different essential oils resonate with you. You'll instinctively be drawn to your favorites. To begin, choose a calming one, such as lavender, chamomile, lemon balm, or patchouli, and a stimulating one, such as peppermint, rosemary, or grapefruit.

Here are some of my favorites of the most popular, safer, and gentler essential oils, along with a brief profile of their qualities and uses in creating a path toward balance. Try them out, or come up with your own list of best scents! I highly recommend delving more deeply into the individual oils on your own or with a professional:

Chamomile (*Anthemis nobilis*): Sweet, herbaceous, and fruity, the Roman variety is anti-inflammatory, anti-allergenic, antiseptic, and astringent. It's great for stress relief, calming the nerves, and, due to its relaxing effect, helps with insomnia. It's often used in treating dry, sensitive, or inflamed skin and also helps with menstrual cramps, headache, earache, arthritis, neuralgia (pain along the course of a nerve), nausea, and more.

Clary sage (*Salvia sclarea*): Herbaceous and lightly sweet, this oil may also have nutty or musky undertones. It's a calming relaxant, good for tension and anxiety, but when fatigue is present, it can energize and invigorate, while reducing blood pressure. This herb is wonderful for women's dream work. Using it in a bedside diffuser before sleep brings not only vivid and lucid dreams but also deeper recall. Have that journal ready! It can also stimulate the body's natural production of estrogen, relieving PMS and preventing hot flashes. It also helps with headaches, coughs, and dry or mature skin. Some consider this soothing scent an aphrodisiac, and others use it to release stuck emotions.

Eucalyptus (*Eucalyptus globulus*): This fresh, powerful scent is antiseptic, and used to fight viruses and bacteria while easing respiratory congestion. Also used with muscle and joint pain, it stimulates blood flow to affected areas. It's a mental stimulant that clears the mind and also alleviates sorrow. Consider it for grieving work.

Frankincense (*Boswellia carterii*): Its woody, spicy, and slightly fruity smell balances and revitalizes the nervous system and stimulates the immune system. Antidepressant and uplifting, it traditionally has been used for spiritual growth and meditation. Excellent for healing breath work, it can help deepen the breath, thus helping your body to calm and center itself. Great for asthma or chest congestion, it can act as an expectorant, soothing congestion while relaxing breathing. It's also used in the care of aging skin.

Geranium (*Pelargonium graveolens*): Sweet and rosy, with fruity and minty undertones. It has anti-inflammatory, antiseptic, astringent, and stimulating properties. It's useful in stress reduction and can be mood enhancing and emotionally uplifting. It can help equalize or balance one's hair *and* skin.

Grapefruit (*Citrus paradisi*): Citrusy (similar to lemon), fresh, light, and slightly sweet, this oil is made from the fruit's rind, and relieves respiratory congestion and revitalizes the spirit. Euphoric and cleansing, it's great for refreshing your environment. It benefits oily or congested skin, improves elasticity, and has diuretic properties. Many citrus oils are phototoxic, including grapefruit, so don't use them if the area of application will be exposed to sunlight within twenty-four hours.

Lavender (*Lavandula augustifolia*): Sweet, balsamic, and herbaceous, this oil is antidepressant, generally relaxing, soothing, and good for insomnia. It has analgesic, antiseptic, and anti-inflammatory properties and can reduce blood pressure, and muscle aches and sprains.

Patchouli (*Pogostemon cablin*): Rich, earthy, and woody, with a note of fruit, this aroma is warm, uplifting, and relaxing. Easing stress, fatigue, and confusion, it's also an aphrodisiac. It's useful for acne; dermatitis; and mature, dry, or chapped skin.

Peppermint (*Mentha piperita*): Uplifting, cooling, and refreshing, this oil is a pain reliever particularly helpful for headaches and migraines. It helps purify and balance, and is excellent for inflammatory skin conditions. Antiseptic and antispasmodic, it's used for colds, flus, and digestive upsets. It also relieves itching and is useful for shock.

Rose absolute (*Rosa damascena*): Deeply floral and sweet (and potentially slightly spicy with nuances of honey), rose oil is one of the most dynamic oils for women. Its calming, supportive energy strengthens a woman's spirit, and its uplifting nature enhances the creative and sexual energies. It's profoundly effective at treating grief, anxiety, and depression. It balances the female hormones, regulates the menstrual cycle, and eases the sensations of PMS and menopause. It gently stimulates circulation and is simply one of the best choices for skin care, especially sensitive, inflamed, and mature or dry skin.

Rosemary (*Rosmarinus officinalis*): Invigorating, woody, and herbaceous, this oil has camphor undertones. A stimulating tonic for mind and body, it's antiseptic, astringent, cleansing, and skin regenerative. It improves blood circulation, and its stimulating qualities make it dynamic for hair and skin care. It can ease mental fatigue and memory loss, as well as muscular aches, strains, and sprains.

Sandalwood (*Santalum album*): Woody, floral, rich, and sweet, this warm, exotic oil is seductive and distinctive. An aphrodisiac, it also aids in meditation and spiritual growth. It relieves stress and can lift depression. It's a tonic for the immune system. It balances dry and oily skin, and is excellent for moisturizing and regenerating the skin.

Vetiver (*Vetiveria zizanioides*): Sweet, earthy, and woody, this antidepressant oil also stimulates the immune system. Given its soothing, relaxing, and anchoring nature, it assists with meditation and grounding when inhaled.

Ylang-Ylang (*Cananga odorata*): Heavy, sweet, floral, and exotic, this oil is antidepressant, antiseptic, aphrodisiacal, and sedative. Both relaxing and stimulating, it's believed to relieve high blood pressure. Coupled with rosemary or lavender, it's excellent for sleep. It's also good for balancing and moisturizing the skin, and can help normalize sebum secretion, but don't use it on sensitive or inflamed skin.

Please heed this note of caution: don't apply undiluted essential oils onto the skin or take oils *internally* without consulting a qualified aromatherapist. If you're pregnant or epileptic, or have liver damage, untreated heart disease, cancer, or any other medical problem, use oils under the proper guidance of a qualified aromatherapy practitioner. The same applies to using oils with children. Always conduct a skin-patch test prior to using an oil for the first time. Apply a small amount of diluted (in a carrier oil) essential oil on the inside of your elbow or behind your ear. Wait twenty-four hours, and if any form of redness or irritation develops, do not use this oil.

Many websites, courses, DVDs, and books provide more opportunities to learn about the more than seven hundred essential oils in existence.

We've explored how your sense of smell and the world of aroma can dramatically affect your memories, emotions, and body. My goal has been to expand your awareness of the value of your olfactory sense and inspire you to take this awareness to a new level in your own experiences. Your sense of smell can bring you great pleasure and healing. Draw it wholly into your consciousness by surrounding yourself with the most organic, natural aromas possible.

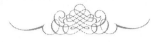

CHAPTER 9

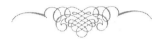

ALL IS RHYTHM

Primordial sound is everywhere as a divine vibration. The ancient Egyptians considered these universal vibratory energies the words of their gods, the Pythagoreans of Greece called them "the music of the spheres," and the ancient Chinese knew them as the celestial energies of perfect harmony. Indeed, every atom in the universe is vibrating. The cosmic symphony is everywhere. We just need to tune in. Mystics, shamans, priests, and healers have heard and helped others hear this symphony for millennia, hence the long and powerful history of using mantras, chanting, toning, drumming, and music to access the balancing and healing nature of sound.

Meditating with a mantra or to the rhythm of your breath brings communion with the divine, toning or chanting your body into attunement brings peace of mind, and drumming restores harmonic patterns of vibration that are in tune with universal vibration, the cosmic symphony. Most of us are now familiar with the quantum physics view that matter is vibrating energy; that is, energy is always on the verge of becoming matter, and matter is always on the verge of becoming energy. How we experience vibration, whether in silence or audibly, can have tremendous impact on our thoughts and thus our mind-body physiology, because thoughts are vibrating energy. Though possibly a new concept for some of you, this is very real. It's what the ancient *rishis*, or sages, tell us in their Vedic texts from five thousand years ago, and now modern science concurs. Many music and sound therapies exist today that help clients attain mental, physical, emotional, or spiritual therapeutic goals.

VIBRATIONAL NUTRITION

When you take in sound vibrations, this energy passes through your middle ear, creating waves in the fluid-filled inner ear, the *cochlea*. These sound waves trigger nerve cells to send electrical energy on to your brain and then through your spine and on to your heart, nerves, and muscles. Your nervous system translates these sound impulses as pleasant (relaxing to the body) or unpleasant (stressful to the body). Aural pleasures, particularly pleasurable music, may enhance our immune-system activity, with our white blood cells picking up this agreeable beat as they flow through the body's lymphatic system. As you listen to enjoyable sounds, endorphins are produced, bathing you in feel-good neuropeptides, or what I like to call "joy juice."

Sound can have amazing effects on delicate cells, tissues, and organs. Vibrating sounds create resonating energy fields around us. When you absorb these energies, they may alter your breath, pulse, blood pressure, muscle tension, skin temperature, brain-wave patterns, and levels of stress hormones in the bloodstream, along with a whole host of other changes to the mind-body physiology.

Naturally, everyone has a different perception of pleasant versus disturbing sounds. What one person hears as symphonic genius is, for another, discordant junk. Pulsing hip-hop may help one person move to the groove with style and efficiency, while for some this music can sound like fingernails across a chalkboard, setting them on edge and making them irritable. Honor your preferences as well as those of others. Be sensitive to how your musical selection may affect those around you.

SOUND ADVICE

Breathing, using mantras, chanting, drumming, and listening to the sounds of nature or music are all ways to bring ourselves to wholeness. Healing sounds resonate within your nervous system, balancing your mind-body physiology. Brain-wave coherence optimizes, and healing chemicals and hormones release within your body. Healing sounds alleviate stress, insomnia, and depression; improve concentration and memory; boost immunity; and reduce pain.

Nature sounds are particularly worth noting because of their profoundly pacifying effect on us. Recall how you feel when listening to early-morning bird melodies, evening cricket chirps, the lonely call of a loon, a haunting wolf's cry, wind rustling through the leaves, a thunderstorm, or a gentle rain—all sounds that enliven and rejuvenate us. (Many nature sounds are available on

CD or downloadable from the Internet if it seems unlikely that a loon or wolf will visit your neighborhood any time soon!) Earth vibrates with life-force energy, and the music of nature can transmit this energy to us.

MUSICAL NOTES

"Music hath charms to soothe the savage beast, to soften rocks or bend a knotted oak," wrote the early-eighteenth-century dramatist William Congreve. And he was right. Music has biochemical effects on the body's biorhythm, the innate, cyclical clock by which all biological systems function. The body's biorhythm conducts all bodily functions, including respiration, circulation, fluid-level regulation, digestion, and detoxification. Music can calm, soothe, or energize these processes, as well as uplift and focus us. Music may reduce pain, tension, and the need for medication. Consider the following effects of various aspects and types of music, which you've probably encountered in your life:

- Faster, louder music produces impulses that increase the heart rate and breathing, while slower, softer music has the opposite effect.

- Sedative music lowers heart and respiration rates along with blood pressure. Slow in tempo with a quality close to the human voice, it tends to feature violins and flutes, as opposed to horns and percussion. Folk music as well as digital or ethereal, otherworldly styles can also be quite sedating.

- The regularity of the beat and the predictability of the harmony and melody also determine whether music wakes you up or puts you to sleep.

- Repetition, such as chanting or drumming, can be very soothing.

- Stimulating music can be quite exhilarating. Mozart (touted for the energy-balancing qualities of his compositions) and Vivaldi are excellent examples.

- The key of the musical piece, whether major or minor, affects your mood. Generally, major melodies convey a happy feeling, while minor ones can evoke sadness.

Sensual Grooves, Organic Rhythms

Easy listening, opera, country, jazz, blues, pop, rock and roll, alternative, Latin, ambient techno, hip-hop, and other musical styles, despite their differences, all have the power to enhance and balance your vitality and energies, and guide your mood and emotional state. Listen to and use them to reflect your present mood or lead your mood to where you wish it to be. You may prefer a dynamic beat at higher volume levels when getting dressed in the morning; soothing and fluid sounds at a moderate tempo in your afternoon at work; and easy, ambient rhythms for winding down in the evening.

The right music can also help ease you into a form of meditation, sound meditation. Sit comfortably with your eyes closed, and breathe in smoothly and evenly, taking in your musical choice. Get into the music with your entire body, mind, and soul. Whether the music is sedating or stimulating in nature, follow your instincts and let the rhythm move you emotionally, physically, spiritually, or in every way.

I enjoy playing music that relaxes me, but at the right time I also enjoy music that gets my body going, for example, the music played in ecstatic dance, which, as mentioned earlier in this book, is a dance where you can move in whatever way feels right to you, becoming one with the music. This is a powerful form of self-healing in which physical activity comes together with music to energize or soothe body and soul.

MEANINGFUL COMMUNICATION

Artful communication, our ability to really hear another person and then share our "voice" with him or her, is such an integral part of our sense of sound and our enjoyment in life. For many, making conversation can be a frightening proposition, especially with a stranger. In the Internet age, with its e-mailing and text messaging, and interaction with machines instead of real people, the art of live chitchat is threatened with extinction. This kind of banter greases the wheels for more meaningful conversation, the kind that creates harmonious relationships. Every great love story, every lifelong friendship, and every major business deal began with that initial conversation. Metaphorically speaking, "finding your voice" and fully expressing it can be incredibly healing for any one of us but especially for the shy wallflower or anyone afflicted with social anxiety. The voice emanates from the throat chakra, our energy center of creative expression or communication. Here are a few simple steps for stimulating more free-flowing conversation:

- Show openness to conversation with a simple statement: "It sure is busy here."

- Introduce yourself in a way that gives the other person enough info to stimulate further questions: "I'm a stay-at-home mom with two toddlers" versus "I work at home."

- Bring up a topic others can relate to: "I saw a great movie last night."

- Associate two different topics to stimulate further conversation: "The theater is next to a wonderful restaurant."

- As your chat winds down, end it gracefully and express thanks: "I need to scoot, but thanks for our chat. I've enjoyed it."

Real Listening

Epictetus the Stoic said, "God gave man two ears but only one mouth, that he might hear twice as much as he speaks." Well said! Certainly, conversation is an art, but one that requires at least two people and a good amount of listening. Monologues have no place off the Shakespearean stage, and dialogue is not about waiting for the other person to take a breath so you can jump in with your lines! Good conversation is give and take. Give your time and attention to the person you're speaking with. If you truly listen, you'll find that many people have fascinating stories to tell. To listen actively, really hearing what another person says, is not only good for your own sense of balance but also is a highly regarded life skill. A good listener can repeat back what the other person has said, with an understanding for the feelings behind the words; for example, "What I heard you say was _____. Is that right?" "You sound as if you're feeling really frustrated." This doesn't mean that you need to immediately grasp everybody's deepest meaning, but a good listener senses when it's time to ask questions—and interesting ones, at that.

Often, some aren't natural and lively conversationalists for one reason: self-absorption. It rears its egotistical head time and again. So instead of trying to beat them, join them! For instance, if the story about how stale the doughnuts were at the staff meeting didn't do it for you, perhaps ask about the doughnuts. Were they jelly filled, glazed, or powdered? Talk about how you're convinced that the devil created gooey, sinfully tempting, glazed doughnuts, and we're all going to hell on a Boston cream pie. Now that'll get the conversational juices flowing! Tangents are just waiting to happen and make for the most interesting exchanges, but you only get there by asking the right questions and really listening.

Consider the following guidelines for effective listening: Try not to edit or hear only what you want to hear. Make eye contact and be present with the other person, instead of daydreaming or thinking of what you want to say while he or she talks. Also resist switching the subject as soon as the other person stops talking. Refrain from relating everything your friend says to your own life or circumstances. Don't be *too* agreeable, nodding your head to everything the person says to avoid conflict, or simply feign interest. Get involved. Be open to what this person shares, and resist arguing or judging. Ultimately, dialogue is about give and take, and communication is an exquisite art form that can be mastered.

Sounding Off

As therapeutic as the sounds of nature and music are, using your voice can be even better for your health than listening. Let's see how vocalization can bring on a harmonious state. Your voice can be a powerful tool for connecting with your inner self, perhaps because your voice box is directly wired into your brain's emotional center. When various emotions surge through us, our speaking voice can suffer. Is it any wonder that a lump in the throat may be the first sign of emotional distress? And just as our emotions can affect our voices, we can also use our voices to affect our emotions. We can vocalize to calm, soothe, balance, or vitalize as needed.

Your voice is not only a tool for expressing yourself but also an excellent vehicle for improving your physical well-being. Singing reduces stress, lowers heart rate, reduces blood pressure, and relieves pain. When we're dealing with highly charged emotional issues, we tend to "go out" of our bodies, whereas singing helps to ground us, to draw us to fully inhabit our bodies. Singing is quite visceral, with the potential to effect great change.

SING IT!

Our voices deliver their own mellifluous melodies outward into the world. When I was a child, I fondly remember my mother's singing. What a happy sound! Go ahead and hum, sing, or shout from the mountaintop; these are all ways to make memories as well as cleanse and strengthen the voice. My pooches are used to my singing on our walks through the forest preserve. I might belt one out in the shower or when driving in my car. Singing can reduce stress and prolong your life. So make a joyful noise—and often!

Whatever song you decide to take on, breathing is the beginning of it all. Breathing diaphragmatically leads to singing that's properly supported by the lower body rather than the throat. This is a well-known secret of the most successful singers. Try this as a good preparatory exercise: relax your jaw, the back of your neck, and your shoulders, and practice inhaling through an imaginary straw and exhaling while making "ssss" sounds.

Personally, I recommend karaoke, which is wildly popular now, and is offered in a wide variety of settings, from sushi bars to lounges to home karaoke units. Try it as a fun and supportive way to explore singing even if you can't carry a tune.

TONING

Toning, an ancient practice now gaining popularity, allows the body to find balance, releasing stress, balancing brain waves, slowing respiration, and actually giving the body a sonic massage from the inside out. This happens through the sustained vibration—like that of a tuning fork—of a sound that resonates through the entire body.

In toning, you sing an elongated vowel sound—such as "ee," "oh," and "ah"—at a certain, comfortable pitch for a prolonged period. The throat is completely open, as is the heart, with no limitation to the sound. Vibrations reverberate through the body, affecting our energy in profound ways, with different sounds working in different ways. Lower "ah" sounds relax the body, while higher "ee" sounds stimulate the brain and wake you up. Simply take in a deep breath and let loose with your tone on the exhalation. Try varying the intensities of tone, sound, and pitch. If you feel constriction or pain anywhere in your body, visualize sending the sound vibration to this area to break up any energy blockage. For best results, try toning every day for at least five to ten minutes per session, and longer if desired. This can be your meditation for the day, if you'd like. The sound becomes your focal point in concentrative meditation.

CHANTING

Chanting also demonstrates the incredible healing powers of the voice. Chants may even be chemically metabolized into "endogenous opiates" that act on the body as both internal painkillers and healing agents. Chanting is similar to toning, but instead you chant a mantra, word, or phrase. Chanting spiritually charged words and sounds can bring about a most harmonizing and spiritual effect; use such words as "shalom," "amen," "Allah," and "om." In yoga philosophy, the Sanskrit sound "om" is believed to be the manifestation of a person's spiritual self. It's a sound of affirmation that allows us to accept who we are. Because I find this to be one of the most resonant sounds for chanting, I end my meditation with it. It's easy to do. Find your comfortable pitch and sing on the exhale, extending the sound for as long as comfortable and repeating as often as you like. Feel the sound vibrate in every fiber of your being, creating a vortex of energy that lifts you to a higher plane of spiritual awareness!

Sounds Of the Chakras

Each chakra corresponds to a particular region of the body and is represented by a unique one-syllable sound called a *bija*, or "seed," mantra. These mantras activate the energy of the chakras to balance and purify the mind and body. Using a bija mantra makes you resonate with the energy of the associated chakra so that you become more aware of your body and its needs. Each sound affects a different facet of well-being, and tuning these centers in this way improves circulation, respiration, and digestion, as well as state of mind, heart, and mood.

In Hatha yoga, the seven healing bija mantras associated with the chakras are:

- "Lam" for the root chakra (base of the spine and tailbone area), which represents our basic survival needs

- "Vam" for the sacral chakra (reproductive organs), which represents biological and creative energy

- "Ram" for the solar plexus chakra (navel area), which is the place from which intentions and desires are manifest

- "Yam" for the heart chakra, the home of compassion and love

- "Ham" for the throat chakra, the center of communication and expression

- "Om" (pronounced "ah-oo-mm") for the third-eye chakra (between the eyebrows), which is the insight center, where we envision fulfillment

- "Ah" for the crown chakra (top of head), where we become aware of our spiritual nature, our connection between individual and universal consciousness

As you chant these sacred sounds, pay attention to the energy patterns that vibrate at each chakra. Listen to this energy more than project a sound onto it. Your chanted vibration melds with the existing vibration in the chakra area to enliven its healing aspects. For example, singing "lam" into your tailbone area might give you a sense of grounding and protective energy. Chanting "yam" to your heart center might surround disturbed emotions with loving-kindness. Chanting "ham" into your throat area might enhance your ability to communicate. Each of you will have your own experience of the bija sounds. Experiment by chanting the sounds on your own.

Sit comfortably with your tailbone drawn toward the earth and your crown to the sky. Lengthen your spine. Take a deep diaphragmatic breath and chant on the exhalation, elongating the "ah" sound. Chant the mantras one at a time, over and over again or in sequence. Gradually, you'll attune to the mantra's finer frequencies until you reach the source energy, where the mantra truly becomes the "seed" of higher consciousness and spiritual energy.

DRUMMING CIRCLE

Once confined to Aboriginal tribes, Native American rituals, or loin-clothed men's circles, drumming has entered the mainstream as a sound therapy. Used by indigenous tribes worldwide for transformation and healing, drumming at certain frequencies brings us to what shamanism refers to as "non-ordinary" reality, where "soul retrieval" takes place. It's where we mentally, physically, emotionally, and spiritually shape-shift.

I conduct drumming circles in wellness settings. Through drumming, a group of people of any age, with or without musical training, focuses on creating rhythm, having fun, and performing stress-relieving exercises. The therapeutic benefits include better concentration, alertness, and physical fitness. It also certainly promotes wellness, happiness, and togetherness.

I belong to a drumming circle, where, together, we create the most amazing and vital energy. It's extraordinary how the individuals in our group respond to each other's rhythms. You don't have to find the rhythm; the rhythm finds you! In this process, the sound of our drums catches us in its spiral, catapulting us into a transformative and breathtaking experience. It just plain brings everyone together into one big, smiley interactive experience.

There are many CDs to help you enjoy and partake of this healing therapy. I highly recommend investing in your own drum! Also consider other forms of instrumental sound to bring harmony into your world, such as Tibetan "singing" bowls, bells, gongs (for a gong bath!—"bathing" in sound in your own environment or in a "gong bath" ceremony offered at yoga studios, and wellness and retreat centers), rattles, wind chimes, and didgeridoo. All of these healing sounds may be used in your environment to anoint, clear, and energize your space.

TOXIC SOUND

Sound levels can be hazardous to our hearing, and in this instance, "sound" refers to noise, and the harm can be both physical and psychological. It's important to take precautions against excessive noise. You can save yourself untold millions of inner-ear cells, plus a lot of aggravation and tension.

If you're around loud noises for extended periods, wear ear-plugs. They're comfortable to wear and made of form-fitting foam, and they come in a variety of colors. I wear them on our many motorcycle trips. Don't worry, you'll hear just fine while wearing them. They only mute the aggressive noises that inflict hearing damage.

The biggest physical concern is that overexposure to loud noise can destroy your ability to hear frequencies above three thousand cycles per second, which robs you of your capacity to enjoy healing music. Optimally, we hear frequencies ranging from twenty to twenty thousand cycles per second, almost ten octaves;

without this capability, music can sound like mush, causing you to miss out on much of the healing energy transmitted by the higher harmonics.

On a purely psychological level, noise undermines our mental and creative energy, distracting us from our focus. Perhaps you're trying to converse with a friend over blaring music or consult with a business associate in a raucous environment, both of which would make communication difficult. Maybe you're trying to enjoy a meal, but a blabbering table-side television takes your attention away from the peas and carrots. A churning air conditioner can prevent you from getting a good night's sleep. All of these little things can cumulatively cause problems.

If the amount of background noise necessitates raising your voice to be heard by someone three feet away, the environment may be hazardous to your hearing. A few sounds and their decibel levels are listed below as a reference. Keep in mind that going up ten decibels doubles the loudness of the sound!

- Wind rustling through the leaves: 20 decibels
- Normal conversation: 50 to 60 decibels
- Hair dryer: 60 to 80 decibels
- Crowded city street: 90 decibels
- Stereo at full volume: 120 decibels
- Jet takeoff: 130 to 140 decibels

Many of you reading this may traipse through a noisy environment every day. Depending on the materials used to construct and decorate your environment (some of which can deaden otherwise intrusive sounds), these sounds can be quite intense. Many companies now manufacture products to lessen noise levels and improve acoustics in a building. These products blend into the environment and go a long way toward moderating "noisy" atmospheres. Here are a few suggestions:

- Wear foam earplugs to suppress noise that can distract and irritate you.

- Look for electronic equipment and appliances that have the lowest possible decibel rating.

- Decorate your environment with soft surfaces such as drapery, upholstery, and carpeting (environmentally friendly, please), all of which absorb noise instead of allowing it to bounce around.

- Install baffles or panels, placing them inconspicuously along walls, hanging them from the ceiling, or putting them under chairs to absorb reverberating sounds.

- Install double-glazed windows (which also helps reduce energy consumption).

- If possible, avoid living or working near a major noise source, such as an airport, a truck route, a freeway, or a busy intersection.

The Deafness Research Foundation is an excellent resource for information related to toxic noise and the harm it can inflict (www.drf.org).

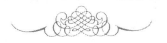

CHAPTER 10

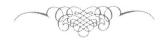

BE THE "VISIONARY"

We've explored how enlightenment, intuition, meditation, creative visualization, and seeing through the mind's eye are integral parts of sight. As we continue our journey toward connecting with inner vision, let's take the concept of sight even further. Keep your eyes wide open. You're about to get some captivating insights into creating better balance and healing within your mind-body physiology.

OUR INNER SIGHT: SEE THE BEAUTY IN EVERYONE

First, let's resist the temptation to judge others based on their outer appearance alone. Our culture is keenly tuned in to how external appearances create specific impressions or emotional responses, which brings to mind the old saying, "What you see is what you get." And our day-to-day interactions can indeed mirror this connection between sight and judgment. Each of us has the ability to see the beauty in ourselves and those around us, which is where our inner sight and emotional intelligence come into play. You have the power to see a person's individual and "soul-full" beauty.

Remember how we positively affirmed our beauty (see chapter 1)? This is the same beauty, the same spirit, that's in everyone and everything. We're all made of the same stuff: recycled earth, water, and air. When you look into the eyes of any living being, see the soul that resides there. This dramatically transforms your interactions and relationships with others, softening hard edges and melting prejudices away.

Try setting your intention to look into the eyes of every person you encounter today: "I intend to look into the eyes of every person I encounter today." Make this a meaningful connection. See the soul that resides in this person. Add a smile if it feels right. Words need not even be said, because this type of heart-to-heart connection is one of the most sublime ways of communicating.

SEE THE LIGHT

Many of us remember the biblical creation story in which God said, "Let there be light." With light, we gained the ability to perceive color, shape, and texture. Our eyes work in such a systematic and routine manner, it's easy to forget the miracle of it all. It's a fascinating process. Our eyes gather light, much like a camera. When we look at something, the retina shoots neurons off to the brain, floating these neurons along an electrochemical stream. The visual cortex in the brain takes this information and makes sense of it, allowing us to define and label what we see. Perhaps 70 percent of all sensory information is taken in through the eyes, where a large number of sense receptors are clustered, which may also be one of the reasons that a quarter of our nutritional intake goes toward feeding our visual apparatus.

Eye Candy

Holistically, the best remedy for eye concerns is to reduce stress, meditate, and relax by taking in the most beautiful of sights. So as you take your post-lunch walk, commute home, or prepare the evening meal, try making it a point to notice only beautiful things. Eventually, you'll run out of conventionally attractive sights and begin finding beauty in the most unexpected places! For instance, as I prepared dinner last night, I found the red pepper on my cutting board particularly appealing and beautiful. I really meditated on that brilliant-red color. When I coupled this with the thought that it was organic and grown without toxic chemicals by a farmer who loves the earth, my appreciation expanded even further. There's a story, and perhaps a bit of bliss, behind everything you can see. Become intimate with these stories. Look for the mystery and sensuality in everything you encounter.

Visualize Beauty

Just as we tend to associate feelings with aromas, we also attach feelings to sights. How you perceive an image can dramatically affect your reaction to subsequent views of the same image or memories of it.

Having traveled to the farthest reaches of the globe, I have some amazing images stored on the ol' hard drive in the noggin. Recalling these sights can bring on a variety of feelings. If a particular image in your mind's eye elicits good feelings, then by all means, go to this place often through visualization. A pristine, pastoral image can induce relaxation and serenity. Familiar images can bring on a sense of peace and comfort. Imagining something you've never seen before can bring on a sense of expansiveness and exhilaration. But disturbing imagery can make you feel stressed, depressed, or ill at ease.

It probably comes as no surprise when I tell you that the hurting world we see through various news media can conjure negative actions and feelings. Consider going on a news fast every so often, separating yourself from the wars, natural catastrophes, and various other atrocities going on around the world. I've done this on numerous occasions, and find it very therapeutic and gratifying.

Also think about the environment you travel through every day. How does it affect you? Is it cluttered, sloppy, and chaotic; or fresh, streamlined, and potent—ripe for your creativity. Remember that your environment is filled with energy, so try to make it a nourishing environment, vibrating with the very best of energy that allows you to transform, enliven, and vitalize every moment of every day. Take pride in creating an environment that surrounds you with this type of transformative energy. Do an inventory of your home and work environments. Do you see, and thus feel, beauty in these spaces? Keep fresh flowers close by, even if it's only one fresh flower in a simple bud vase. Consider the colors that surround you. Think of beautiful sights that please you. Now consider a few insightful ways to beautify your environment, whether this means making updates or repairs, or adding simple, joyful touches.

COLOR YOUR WORLD

Color affects our health, mood, and way of thinking. You may prefer one color over another because of how it makes you feel. As a matter of fact, your preference for a certain color may indicate that your body needs it. The pleasant response your body gives to a certain color is a thank-you from your energy system. In the spa world, many have integrated color therapy (also called *chromatherapy*) into their services. This therapy is used to maintain or change bodily vibrations through visualization, colored light, color-therapy massage, or hydrotherapy treatments. Of course, there's also the matter of how color can influence energy flow and activity throughout a space. Color therapy is now used for its therapeutic value in a variety of settings, from hospitals to schools to prisons. We'll cover this further shortly, but for now let's just say that color, regardless of intensity, has great power.

Light is absorbed by the eyes and converted into another form of energy, which enables us to see color. This energy affects us, and remarkably, even people without sight feel it. Light energy stimulates the pineal and pituitary glands, regulating hormones and many other physiological systems. As electromagnetic energy, color can profoundly affect our energy fields, creating changes in the mind and body. The colors we see are part of the visible electromagnetic spectrum of light that radiates from the sun. This spectrum ranges from the longest-wavelength color, red, which vibrates at a low, dense frequency, to the shortest-wavelength color, violet, which vibrates at the highest frequency. In between are the colors orange, yellow, green, blue, and indigo. Each of these colors vibrates at its own frequency, and together these colors possess the power to heal and balance on many levels, because we sense color vibration through not only our vision but also all of our physical systems and organs. Everything responds to these color frequencies, which is why color therapy so profoundly affects us, creating balance and facilitating healing.

The Right Hues for Your Many Moods

Here are some interesting tidbits about color and its effects on us and our environment:

Red stimulates and excites, warming the body, and increasing heart rate, respiration, and brain-wave activity, which is why those with high blood pressure or hypertension should refrain from too much red in their environments. However, mothers are encouraged to dangle mobiles with red, shiny balls over their infants, because it stimulates their brain activity. Restaurants use red to stimulate the appetite (orange also). Red is discouraged in the bedroom, because despite its ability to stimulate lovemaking, it can hinder sound slumber.

Orange not only stimulates the appetite but also reduces fatigue. So if there are any finicky eaters in the household, try using an orange tablecloth. But, of course, if you're on a diet, avoid orange. Interestingly, orange also stimulates people to buy.

Yellow is a happy color! Its stimulating qualities can help a failing memory, so visualize a brilliant yellow next time you've forgotten a date or name or lost your keys. It also raises blood pressure and pulse rate but not as much as red does.

Green is the color of nature, reminding us of spring and new beginnings. It nurtures hopeful feelings, and has a soothing, relaxing effect on the mind-body physiology. Green also counters anxiety connected to controlling impulsive and excessive eating. Perhaps that avocado-green fridge isn't so bad after all!

Pink is a very soothing color, promoting peaceful emotions, and even relaxing the muscles. Its tranquilizing effect is effectively used in hospitals, prisons, and drug-rehab centers.

Blue is also quite the relaxing color. No wonder it works so well in the bedroom; it brings on sound slumber and pleasant dreams. Its calming effect lowers blood pressure, respiration, and heart rate. It also has a cooling effect on hot days. Also, classrooms are sometimes painted blue to calm kids who are prone to tantrums or aggressive behavior.

Seeing Colors

Now let's take a closer look at the power of color. As I define each color's effect on us, I relate it to the chakra system, or what's called the "energy system" in the medical paradigm. As mentioned in chapter 6, there are seven major energy centers, or *chakras*, within us. Each chakra is a vortex of energy, a spiritual opening in the body where subtle energies can enter and leave. Chakras process subtle energy and convert it into chemical, hormonal, and cellular changes in the body. The chakras act as doorways to our consciousness, allowing ethereal energy to become physical energy, and physical energy to return to the ethereal realm.

To positively affect the chakras with color, surround yourself with the colors for the healing you seek. It may be a matter of an overall chakra "tune-up." Wear, eat, and breathe these colors into your body for healing. Before we get down to the nitty-gritty, remember this synopsis: warm and bright reds, oranges, and yellows stimulate, giving energy and strength. Greens and blues cool, soothe, cleanse, and balance. Muted oranges, yellows and golds, deep purple, and indigo calm anxiety and restlessness. Purple induces lightness of being and enhances intuition.

As you read on and become more familiar with each color, think of ways to integrate more or less of a particular color into your world. For instance, if you feel you need help with your fifth chakra, in the throat area—the seat of our ability to communicate—then bring as much blue into your life as possible. Eat blueberries, wear blue jeans, look at the brilliant day-blue sky, gaze at the indigo nighttime sky, paint your walls blue, and consider accessorizing your surroundings with blue. And importantly, when you visualize, color the images you see with lots of healing blue!

Red is traditionally the color of the root chakra, located at the base of the spine. In its highest manifestation, red expresses divine will, because the root chakra is at the center of our survival. Red vitalizes and stimulates. It's responsible for a sound physical body, because it affects our circulatory system, digestion, and elimination. When these systems aren't working harmoniously, you might feel tremendous fatigue. Red helps maintain the skin's color, and gives energy to nerve tissue and bone marrow. A lack of red can manifest as abscesses, anemia, blood disorders, cancer, and insomnia, as well as circulatory, digestive, and heart problems.

Orange is traditionally the color of the sacral chakra, seen as the center of fertility, both creative and sexual. Orange expresses wisdom in its greatest form, and gives energy and strength to the sex organs. Orange can also relieve depression brought on by insecurity and fear, and can build self-esteem through creative and intellectual stimulation. Some illnesses associated with a lack of orange's vibratory energy are asthma, epilepsy, female reproductive problems, kidney ailments, and mental instability.

Yellow is traditionally the color of the solar-plexus chakra, expressing the divine intellect, because this chakra is where you form opinions based on all subtle energetic levels of sensation. These sensations and your reactions to them allow you to develop a strong sense of self. Yellow works with the body as a purifier and cleanser. It illuminates and inspires, allowing your higher consciousness to develop. It promotes all forms of mental activity, and also stimulates optimism. Some illnesses associated with a lack of yellow energy include skin diseases, heartburn, hemorrhoids, diabetes, and impotence.

Traditionally the color of the heart chakra, green is the universal color for healing. It's quite balancing and cleansing, and brings energy and happiness to our center of unconditional love, the heart. Green creates a condition of well-being and stability on all levels, helping overcome anxiety, intolerance, and irritability.

Work with the color green if you're challenged with any of the following afflictions: cancer, miscarriage, nervous disorders, blood pressure and circulatory problems, heart disease, gallstones, and kidney stones.

Blue is traditionally the color of the throat chakra, and expresses truth, because the fifth chakra deals with outward expression of self, the way we tactfully and elegantly communicate with others. Blue works primarily with the throat energies in that it expresses creativity in a way that reflects the inner self. Bring more blue into your mind-body physiology if you find yourself challenged by eye, ear, nose, and throat problems, as well as irritability, laryngitis, tonsillitis, and sexual dysfunction.

Indigo is traditionally the color of the third-eye chakra, and expresses enlightenment, which is the ability to see things as they really are, thus promoting clarity in thought as well as tolerance. Indigo purifies the bloodstream and mental processes, and also promotes unity and stability of your higher subtle bodies. It has even been used to induce local and, in certain cases, total anesthesia. Lack of indigo is said to result in mental instability; lung ailments; menopausal problems; sterility; delirium; and eye, ear, and nose problems.

Violet is traditionally the color of the crown chakra, and can create incredible lightness of being in the body while helping to open the doors of perception. It expresses metamorphosis and devotion while enhancing inspirational energies and intuition. Violet encourages dedication to higher truths and ideals by blending the love in the color red with the truth and devotion in the color blue. Bring more violet into your life if you find yourself challenged by scalp problems, blood ailments, tumors, vertigo, concussion, delusional disorders, or convulsions.

This has been a brief overview of color therapy and its beneficial effects on your mind-body physiology. Please take it upon yourself to study further this intriguing and provocative subject.

Fresh, vital, and beautiful, the language of our senses is universal, and is revealed to us in the precious details. May your senses gather you and bring you home, where you can experience your truest whole self.

CHAPTER 11

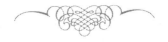

THE BODY BEAUTIFUL

Having explored returning to our senses as a practice for connecting with consciousness (see chapters 7 through 10), now let's look at some more practical aspects of caring for our sense organs. These are conscious-care rituals that further provide body bliss.

THE SKIN WE'RE IN

Skin truly connects us with life, because we first begin the experience of touch through our skin. I've encouraged you to think of the sensations your skin allows you to delight in, whether it's touching or being touched. We've shared rituals for connecting with consciousness and pleasure healing through the skin, such as a self-massage and a luxurious aromatherapy bath. The full range of life's experiences is projected onto and held deep within your skin's surface. Your skin is this and so much more.

As the sense organ of touch, let's look at skin in its unabashed nakedness. Your skin is your body's largest organ, weighing from 6 to 12 pounds. Your skin busily sheds over a million cells every hour. A single square centimeter of skin contains 200 nerve endings, 100 sweat glands, 15 oil glands, 10 hairs, 2 cold receptors, and 25 pressure-sensing receptors. Our skin shields us from rain, snow, and sunshine, and protects us with a constant bath of moisture and natural oils. A primary organ for excreting toxins, it breathes in oxygen and expels carbon dioxide, and regulates body temperature. It's also involved in metabolizing and storing fat. Exposed to sunlight, it produces life-essential vitamin D.

Be meticulous in caring for your skin—all of it! Remember, as your body's largest organ, your skin reflects so many choices you make each and every day toward your well-being. It *will* reflect your lifestyle. A consistent, holistic regimen of cleansing, toning, moisturizing, exfoliating, and protecting with organic skin-care products is a good beginning. When combined with stress management, good nutrition, physical activity, adequate hydration, and healthful lifestyle choices, such as moderating sun exposure and not smoking, your skin will radiate a profound well-being and beauty.

The Nature of Skin

How's this for a "beauty-licious" visualization? Healthy skin is alive with vibrating energy. It's radiant, smooth, supple, elastic, and moist. It has a slight flush to it from optimal blood circulation. Antioxidants are hard at work, hormones are balanced, and stress is under control. Oil and sweat glands intelligently and lovingly bathe your skin with just the right amount of natural oil and moisture, which maintains the skin's natural acid mantle. All the while, your healthy, radiant skin is in a constant state of renewal, turning over and shedding skin cells in a sort of healthful internal dance. Every cell in your body communicates and works harmoniously. This is synergy in motion.

While this wonderful balance is indeed how your skin wants to react, you can damage this balance by putting your skin in harm's way. However, you can minimize external damage by examining everything you do, which is sometimes easier said than done, since many people don't even realize that routine activities damage their skin. The perfectly natural ways to create beautiful skin are to reduce stress, eat healthfully, stay hydrated, get a good balance of exercise and rest, follow a healthful skin-care regimen with pure products, practice sun protection, and avoid smoking. And naturally, always use a gentle massaging motion when manipulating your skin. Rough tugging, rubbing, or abrasive handling with your fingers, towels, tissues, or machines damages your skin. Look for 100 percent natural and organic cotton fiber tissues.

Get Naked

Nakedness is an age-old metaphor for being spiritually open, the idea being that it's unnecessary to hide your true essence from others. So I heartily suggest getting a healthy dose of nakedness every day. Go face to face with your skin. Sleep naked, drink your morning coffee in the buff, and even make a couple of business calls (warning: only try this one at home!). As you become oh so comfortable in the skin you're in, you're more apt to notice changes in skin texture, lumps, or bumps that may require further attention.

Caring for Our Skin

I recommend indulging in regular facial treatments with a skin-care professional. They can set you on the proper path toward blissful, skin-type appropriate, organic skin care. Minimally, the change of seasons is a particularly good time, because your skin usually changes to adapt to climate changes. And it's delightful to put your skin in someone else's capable, healing hands.

Skin-care specialists are well versed in basic skin-care techniques. Naturally, the world of the spa offers a number of progressive, specialty skin-care treatments, but following are some steps you can take on your own. You can adapt these basic steps to your skin type, and the product and application depend on whether you're working on facial or body skin:

1. **Cleanse:** Wash your skin with a gentle cleansing agent to remove dirt and oil, and balance the skin—gently, please! Be extra gentle on your face and neck. Use upward and outward strokes. Around the delicate upper-eye area, work from the inner corner out; around the lower-eye area, work from the outer corner in. Masks can deeply cleanse pores and reduce their size, with some masks serving double duty as exfoliants.

2. **Tone:** Apply a clarifying liquid to firm skin tissue, reduce pore size, and remove cleanser residue. Mist it on or apply it with a cotton pad. Look for toners with botanicals, herbs, and essential oils. (I love my homemade rosewater!)

3. **Moisturize:** Apply hydrating lotions, creams, butters, and oils that are humectant (draws moisture into the skin), emollient (preserves moisture already in the skin), and lubricating (lays a thin, protective layer on the outside of the skin). Apply to damp skin to lock in extra moisture. Don't use heavy, greasy creams. Your skin needs to breathe! Lightly pat moisturizer around your eye area with the pad of your middle or index finger.

4. **Exfoliate:** Apply exfoliants to remove the top, dead layers of skin cells and debris to encourage better cell turnover and prevent clogged pores. But please, moderation is key. Exfoliating too often or with products that are too strong can strip away the skin's natural acid mantle, throwing your skin into an imbalanced state. Always follow product label instructions.

5. **Protect:** Adhering to the above four techniques ultimately provides vital protection of our skin, encouraging healthy skin-cell turnover; safeguarding the skin's natural acid mantle; and helping maintain the skin's natural strength, elasticity, and resiliency. Be sure to use sun protection. As healthy as sunbathing

in moderation can be for our health, unprotected sun exposure is a prime cause of wrinkles, and 90 percent of skin cancers are from sun damage.

Protecting the Skin Barrier

The most important goals in organic skin care are to encourage regular sloughing off and turnover of skin cells, and maintain the skin's natural acid mantle, which is a combination of sebum and perspiration that your body secretes to moisturize your skin's surface. Achieving these goals can protect and help rebuild damaged collagen and elastin (chief protein in your skin's elastic fibers) to maintain skin strength, elasticity, and resiliency. Several important methods optimize cellular turnover, from the inside out and the outside in. Body brushing, cleansing with a facial mitt or buff, using deeply cleansing masks, and using alpha hydroxy acids, or AHAs (natural, organic fruit acids), can all help exfoliate dead surface cells and maintain efficient skin-cell turnover. Your skin can get AHAs through a variety of treatments, from peels to moisturizing lotions. To protect your skin's natural acid mantle, which covers your entire body, use gentle acid-balanced cleansers to wash. Avoid antibacterial or deodorant soaps, which tend to be harsh.

The Organic and Sacred

Just as all mindful practices create a fertile medium for your exquisite growth as an individual in body, mind, and spirit, your selection of beauty or personal-care products is important for your well-being. I like to think of these lotions and potions, sprays and balms, oils and elixirs as food for the skin. Products placed on our skin have direct entrée to the bloodstream, whereas the food we ingest is first metabolized by the liver. Ensure that the "food" for your skin is as pure, organic, and devoid of toxins as possible. This is no small feat, because many personal-care and household-cleaning products are rife with potentially carcinogenic, endocrine-disrupting, and allergenic ingredients. Become a mindful label reader, and know as much as you can about not only what you put *into* your body but also what you put *on* it.

The exciting news is that the marketplace has grown prolifically to offer natural and organic products that are pure goodness, while providing high-quality education about these products conveying why they're so good for our beauty and well-being. Whether the food we eat, or the products we use on our body or in our environment, elegantly formulated products contain a synthesis of botanicals, whole foods, and, most certainly, *certified*-organic and biodynamic plants (flowers, herbs, grains, fruits, vegetables, and more) that breathe and germinate within soil that's potent with the life force. Humming with good vibrations, this soil grows the finest of fruits, and the finest of fruits makes for the finest body and mind. Together, let's ground ourselves in this nourishing energy that can transform, enliven, and vitalize our every moment of every day. Again, what a great visualization and positive affirmation!

Being the "mother organica" that I am, I'll always point you to certified-organic products. Many claims for natural (and even organic!) products are less than truthful, using petroleum-based and potentially toxic ingredients synthesized in laboratories, hence the extra importance of organic certification.

Remember that using organic and biodynamic ingredients from the natural world nurtures the most vibrant flow of prana (life-force energy) through our bodies (and the earth). The integrity and wholeness in certified-organic and biodynamic plant products—the high level of vitamins, minerals, essential fatty acids, amino acids, phytosterols, enzymes, natural sugars, and more—provide a vital spectrum of benefits for the mind, body, skin, scalp, and hair. They cleanse, purify, hydrate, detoxify, stimulate, soothe, smooth, and protect, using the energy and intelligence from food grown in rich, fertile soil.

PLEASURE-HEALING RITUAL: Give Beauty to Yourself and Others

Whether you're caring for yourself or giving a treatment to a loved one, massaging, cleansing, toning, moisturizing, exfoliating, protecting your skin, shampooing, shaving, giving a hand massage, or bathing, use conscious care. Every time you care for your body in any way, make it a scared ritual (review the self-massage in chapter 7).

During any of the above treatments, close your eyes and come inside, becoming "centered" in self. Breathe smoothly and deeply, setting your intention to be fully present. Give loving attention and send healing energy to yourself, experiencing every nuance of the treatment. Use loving, intuitive touch when stroking your body, skin, or hair. Thoughtfully choose the products to use on your body or release into the water or air. Feel the textures and smell the aromas. Feel the layers of your skin under your fingers, sensing every nuance of this process and this time spent nurturing yourself.

By the way, did you know that deep breathing is a face-friendly activity? The skin directly uses about 7 percent of the oxygen we inhale, which is another great reason for regular physical activity. You'll simply glow!

OUR CROWNING GLORY

As an extension of the skin, our hair deserves mention, coupled with our scalp, because they live in such harmony when healthy. Hair is one of the most exquisite fibers found in nature. As our "crowning glory," when consciously cared for, our hair is lustrous, resilient, supple, and strong—in essence, healthy.

Healthy hair begins with a healthy body and mind. Optimal nutrition, adequate physical activity, and minimization of stress (physical, mental, emotional, and environmental) are key to maintaining healthy skin, hair, and nails. Additionally, mechanical (such as rough treatment, excessive pulling, wringing, or heat), environmental, and chemical stressors can greatly compromise the hair's integrity.

A luxurious, nurturing hair and scalp bath is an integral part of holistic self-care. Who wouldn't want to stay at that shampoo bowl indefinitely while a beauty professional shampoos or massages her scalp? This is pleasure and healing personified! The scalp is an area rich in nerves and blood supply. Slowly and gently massaging the scalp improves blood circulation to the head, while relaxing muscles and nerves. This helps refresh the mind and body, while relieving tension and fatigue, because of the fresh oxygen and glucose supply to the brain and spinal cord, along with the increase of hormones and enzymes necessary for brain growth and relaxation of the body. And let's not forget about the healing power of scalp massage for delivering a fresh blood and nutrient supply to the hair papilla, or root, nurturing hair growth.

Massage your scalp to calm, cleanse, purify, detoxify, soothe, and energize, while nourishing, moisturizing, and strengthening with the purest of plant ingredients in your product choices. Hair and scalp are transformed, silkened, smoothed, soothed, and protected, becoming simply radiant. Spend several minutes in this sacred ritual. Be in the moment and luxuriate in the process. Give yourself every bit of your loving attention. Massage your scalp in small, rotary motions using the pads of your fingertips. Work from your forehead to your crown, your side hairline to your occipital area, and the hairline behind your ears to the center nape. Be sure to massage your entire scalp. (If you're doing a hair bath or conditioner treatment, rinse thoroughly, preferably under filtered water.) Visualize increasing the blood flow to your scalp. Visualize sending freshly oxygenated blood to your brain. Visualize increasing the flow of the life-force energy through your mind-body physiology, while fully taking in this silky, sensuous, fragrant massage for your scalp and hair. Experience the inner peace and the outer beauty.

SEE THE BEAUTY IN EYE CARE

Our vision is indeed priceless! Look all around you right now. Realize the wonderful gift you have in your ability to visually take in your world. Don't take your vision for granted. Over time, eyestrain, stress, exposure to environmental toxins, lack of exercise, inadequate or inappropriate nutritional intake, and simply neglect can lead to large and small woes, such as presbyopia, glaucoma, cataracts, and macular degeneration. Yes, some of these conditions have genetic components, but this only means that you need to be even more diligent in caring for your magnificent peepers. Begin caring for your eyes by practicing stress reduction and meditation, and viewing beautiful visual treats, real or imagined, all of which are of paramount importance for resting your mind and, in turn, your eyes.

Take It Easy on Your Eyes

You can also protect your eyesight by concentrating on certain eye-care practices. Get regular eye exams, lots of exercise, and plenty of rest, and give maximum attention to proper nutrition. Did you know that more than 25 percent of the nutrients we absorb from our food go to our visual system? Take care to rest your eyes, hydrate them with natural eyedrops or tears as needed, use only the most natural products in and around your eyes, and reduce exposure to environmental allergens and toxins. Exercise your eyes by consciously blinking, rotating them, and alternately focusing them on close and distant objects. Consider programmed vision therapy or eye calisthenics to maintain your eyesight, or if you find your vision worsening. Alone or in combination, these practices can strengthen your body's natural ability to avert eyestrain and eyesight deficiencies, as well as wrinkled skin, puffiness, and dark circles around the eyes.

Eye Yoga

Doing eye exercises and massage every day can help relax, cleanse, and strengthen your eyes. As for eye exercise, routinely move the muscle surrounding the eye's lens (the ciliary muscle) and those surrounding the eyeball (the extraocular muscles) in different directions. Every one of my yoga classes includes a bit of "eye yoga." As my students move into certain postures, I ask them to stretch their eyes as far as they can toward the sky and the back wall, from side to side, and so on. The many small vessels and muscles surrounding the eyes can benefit from increased blood flow and prana (life force energy) just as much as the rest of the body. Also consider the following:

- At intervals throughout the day, focus on objects at varying distances to strengthen the muscles used to focus your eyes and to give your eyes a break. Try this simple exercise: hold a finger about a foot away from your face, at nose level, and focus on it for ten seconds. Now shift your focus to an object about ten feet away, again focusing for ten seconds. This is one round; do ten rounds of this exercise, and then relax. Do this several times throughout the day.

- To relax your optic nerve, enhance blood circulation, and relieve muscular tension in and around your eyes, tighten your eye muscles by squeezing your eyes tightly shut, and then gently open your eyes, letting tension dissolve away. Blink several times as you turn your head from side to side. "Palm" your eyes by briskly rubbing your palms together and then gently cupping them over (but not touching) your closed eyes and nose. For an extra treat, add a drop of your favorite essential oil to your palms before rubbing them together. Relax and pay attention to your breathing for a few moments. Do these practices several times a day.

- Treat yourself to daily serenity checks, where you soften and relax your facial features by gently closing your eyes and consciously letting your muscles relax (what a great mindfulness trigger!), without furrowing the brow, frowning, or scrunching the eyes tightly. Just letting all the muscles hang is a very conscious way to witness any tension held in the face and body so you can choose to release these held tensions. It's not so much an exercise as a serenity check-in.

- Massage the eye area using an organic oil like sweet-almond oil. With your ring fingers, gently press around your eye socket from the outer corner, along the bottom edge, and then along the top of your eyelid, just below the brow bone. Repeat several times, preferably at bedtime.

Actively caring for your eyes with these practices will make them work more efficiently so that they exhibit less deterioration with age. Many of us take a passive approach to our eyes, simply relying on corrective lenses to solve vision problems. Because a whole world of visual therapies is available, now we can take a proactive approach to protecting our eyesight.

Eye Nourishment

In traditional Chinese medicine, the eyes are said to be nourished by the liver. The liver meridian runs through tissues surrounding the eyes, bringing the life-force energy to this entire area. The liver filters many of the toxins we take in, so it's essential to eat as healthfully as possible (lots of veggies and fruits!) to support the liver's vital function of processing toxins we're exposed to.

Milk thistle is one of the best herbs to detoxify the system, cleanse the blood, and support liver function. Also consider burdock and dandelion in whole-food, tea, or tincture form. The herbs eyebright and bilberry specifically support eye health. Find any of these at your favorite health or whole-foods store.

Also, as a preventive measure against glaucoma and cataracts, and to protect the general health of your eyes, reduce your intake of saturated fat and cholesterol, which can block the tiny vessels surrounding the eyes, resulting in arteriosclerosis.

Soothing Eye Treatments

Consider one of the following natural eye treatments, each of which, when applied over closed eyes for fifteen to twenty minutes, serves a delicious and soothing purpose. Now I'm not a huge proponent of multitasking, but consider one of these treatments while you're relaxing, napping, meditating, doing visualization, or taking a bath:

- Cotton pads doused with ice-cold organic milk or rosewater and placed over your closed eyes (especially in the morning) help reduce puffiness and soothe irritated or bloodshot eyes.

- Placing cucumber, apple, or potato slices over your closed eyes has the same effect.

- Cooled black tea, chamomile, and calendula, in bags or compresses, soothe and reduce swelling. To make a compress, put two tablespoons of the tea or herb into a cup of water, boil, cool, and strain. Dip cotton pads or a washcloth into the tea and place over your closed eyes. Relax as long as time permits, the longer the better.

You Look Marvelous

Be exceptionally careful about what you put in or around your eyes, such as makeup or contact lenses. Your eyes are extremely sensitive, and a bit of conscious care up front can prevent all sorts of problems later, such as nasty bacterial infections or allergic reactions.

- If you wear contacts, consider using a natural, preservative-free contact lens solution, available at most stores that carry organic products.

- Be careful with eye makeup, throwing out any that's six months old; discarding after three months is even better. Look for hypoallergenic, natural, and organic eye makeup.

- Use organic almond, olive, or jojoba oil to gently massage the eye areas. Also use these oils on a dampened cotton pad to gently remove makeup.

- Each night, use a cotton swab to brush a light application of olive or castor oil along your brows and lashes. Over time this creates thicker, more-lustrous lashes and brows.

- Always wear sunglasses with ultraviolet protection when you're in bright sunlight.

- Don't smoke! Smoking creates deep wrinkles around your eyes and mouth.

See the Light: Healthy Lighting

We need to see the light—literally. Certain people suffer dearly when they don't get enough light. Tied to our circadian rhythms, this problem especially concerns individuals who miss out on daylight by working the night shift. Endless rainy days and jet lag also bring on light-deprivation woes. At the most serious level, certain individuals who don't get enough daylight (especially during winter months, when daylight hours diminish, or in northern latitudes, where darkness prevails for lengthy periods) experience a condition called SAD, or seasonal affective disorder, which can cause fatigue, irritability, and depression. Exposure to bright light from a specially designed light box available in specialty stores and catalogs, or through holistic physicians, can treat the condition.

It's important to get up with the sun, do as much as possible during normal daylight hours, and let your body enjoy plenty of natural light. Natural light helps normalize adrenal function and, more specifically, cortisol (the stress hormone) levels, and also triggers essential physiological processes involving the nervous and endocrine systems. In addition, it greatly enhances metabolization of vitamin D, the sunshine vitamin, which stimulates calcium absorption and the building of strong bones, and is an important nutrient in fighting several cancers.

Bringing your life into rhythm with the ebb and flow of natural light is pretty straightforward. Perform as many of your daily activities as possible in natural or full-spectrum lighting. Full-spectrum lighting will bring out the truest colors in your surroundings, ease eyestrain, reduce fatigue, and help improve your mood. Try to get at least fifteen to twenty minutes of sunlight every day. And here's an interesting notion: yogis say that gazing at a full moon strengthens your eyesight and your heart. So go ahead; commune with the man in the moon!

THE NOSE KNOWS

We've explored holistic pleasure-healing approaches that involve our sense of smell and discussed emotional connections made with the nose, but your nose also possesses great physical powers. As you breathe in and out, mucous membranes block bacteria and dust particles from entering the body. Nose hairs warm the air entering your lungs and prevent a perpetual runny nose by keeping mucous secretions toward the back of your throat. To keep these natural processes happening, it's important to build an immune system capable of staving off head colds or sinusitis. When the inevitable stuffy nose comes your way, using a vaporizer with eucalyptus, juniper, or tea tree essential oil can help clear things up. However, if you're plagued by nasal polyps, a deviated septum, or any other malady that prevents you from breathing normally through your nose, seek medical attention. Also review the dynamic effects of aromatherapy on your health and beauty in chapter 8.

PLEASURE-HEALING RITUAL: Nasal Irrigation—Clearing the Way for Optimal Breathing

As an educator of mind-body health and Ayurveda, I not only regularly teach but also personally practice *nasal irrigation*, also called "nasal lavage" or "sinus rinsing," a practice that can purify and revitalize the breathing passages; reduce allergies; and fight colds, congestion, sinus problems, asthma, and other respiratory ills. It's an easy, low-tech way to wash out viruses, bacteria, mold, allergens, dust, mucus, and the general crud that lands inside the nose and sinus passages, including natural chemicals called *cytokines*, which promote inflammation. Remove the mucus, and you remove the inflammation. It's also great to do it preflight to keep your breathing passages moist. Some hear "nasal irrigation" and say, "Doesn't sound too pleasant to me!" But trust that the end result makes this quite the pleasure-healing practice.

Several products are on the market for nasal irrigation, but the *neti pot* is the most common. Long used among the yoga set and now widely available, it's a small container with a spout. Here are brief instructions for using it:

(1) Make an isotonic solution (the same saltiness as body fluids) by mixing eight ounces of purified or distilled water (room temperature or warm) with a quarter teaspoon of salt, and a quarter teaspoon of baking soda (which keeps the solution from stinging) in the neti pot; (2) Tilt your head sideways. (I actually tilt my whole body slightly sideways.) The key is to get the water to travel far enough up the nasal cavity to come back around the other side. Place the spout up into the nostril (which is positioned higher) as far as it will go comfortably, and slowly pour the warm saltwater. The water will run out the other nostril. Repeat on the other side. You may want to gently blow your nose in between and after this process.

I do this procedure in the shower in the morning, because it's easy to let the excess water just go down the drain, but you can certainly do it over the sink. Not only will you end up with clear sinuses (quite blessed, this!), but you'll also be able to draw in the deepest, most healing breath possible.

Another technique, called *nasya* in Ayurveda, is synergistic when used in combination with the neti pot but can also be done on its own. It involves the application of a few drops of oil to the nasal membranes to keep them lubricated and moist. The oil should be an edible (preferably organic) grade of olive, sweet almond, or sesame. You can also use herbal aromatic oils containing small amounts of camphor, eucalyptus, and menthol. Place a drop or two on your little finger and apply inside the nostril. Gently sniff, and then repeat on the other side. Repeat several times during the day or as required.

SOUND HEALTH

Along with increasing exposure to soothing sounds, practicing sound therapies, and reducing damage-inducing noise levels, here are a few commonsense, but often overlooked, ways to protect your ears:

- Eat a low-fat, low-cholesterol diet. A high-fat diet clogs and hardens the arteries, impairing the flow of nutrient-rich blood throughout the body, including to the inner ear.

- Get regular exercise to improve blood circulation.

- If you experience any degree of hearing loss, get your hearing checked by a medical professional. Your problem may be as simple as wax buildup, or it could be more serious. Other hearing problems

> requiring immediate attention include ringing in the ears, vertigo, and TMJ (temporomandibular joint) problems.

- Consider decreasing your cell phone usage, using ear buds, or putting an electromagnetic phone shield on it. Some concern has been raised about how cell phones send out electromagnetic frequencies that travel into the brain through the ear canal, potentially causing cancer.

- Be extremely gentle when cleansing the ear and ear-canal area. Also be sure to include the ears in your delicious self-massage, massaging gently with a small amount of oil. Pull on your earlobe, and then delicately massage entirely around it with your thumb and index finger. Use the tip of the index finger to gently massage behind the ear and around the ear opening, without going into the ear canal. This simple process relaxes the muscles and joints in the jaw and neck, and also stimulates many organs and glands, especially those affecting the skin.

Naturally, check with your doctor about any persistent problems with your ears or hearing, but consider the following natural therapies, especially with an earwax buildup or persistent ear infections:

- Using an eyedropper, put a couple of drops of hydrogen peroxide in each ear. Gently rinse each ear with a bulb syringe filled with warm water. Do this once a day for a couple of days.

- Lie on your side and place ten drops of warm organic sesame oil in your ear canal. Pull your earlobe down to let the oil flow in. Rest in this position for five minutes, and then place a cotton ball in your ear, turn over, and repeat on the opposite side. Finish by lying on your back for a few minutes. Do this treatment in the early morning but not more often than once a year. (Never put anything in your ear if you believe your eardrum may have burst.)

- Reduce your intake of stimulants such as caffeine, tobacco, alcohol, aspirin, and tonic water, which are all thought to aggravate hearing problems.

SINK YOUR TEETH INTO THIS

While our ears are the sense organs for hearing sound, our mouths are the sense organs for delivering sound. We've explored how the mouth is home to our sense of taste and the foundation of the digestive process. The ten thousand taste buds across the broad expanse of your tongue distinguish sweet, sour, salty, pungent, bitter, and astringent flavors. The mouth, lips, teeth, gums, and tongue are quite sensual parts of the body. Your tongue allows you to communicate with your world. Your lips are a provocative extension of the mucous membranes inside the mouth. Your teeth express happiness and pleasure when you flash your pearly whites.

Your gums hold and support your teeth. Lavish your mouth with loving attention. Slather organic balms on your lips, eat nourishing foods, meticulously cleanse your mouth, massage your gums every day with a bit of organic sesame or sweet-almond oil, and sing a happy tune!

Dental services have become a mainstay in the spa realm, and the more holistic the better. There are actually a number of "eco-dental wellness" spas where you can discover your inner and outer smile.

Lip Service

Our highly sensitive lips contain specialized sensors near the skin's surface that respond to the slightest stimulation. Gently rub the pad of your index finger across your closed lips, and then rub the skin on your cheek. Feel the difference? It's quite dramatic, isn't it? These sensors are found in just a few places on the body: the lips and tongue, palms of the hands, soles of the feet, nipples, clitoris, and penis, which is why a kiss is never just a kiss but an abiding symbol of emotional connection and love.

Unlike the rest of your skin, your lips have no melanin to protect them and no oil glands, which can contribute to potential lip problems, such as burning, chapping, and dryness. To protect your lips, try the following:

- Drink plenty of pure water to keep your lips moisturized from the inside out. Limit alcohol and caffeine, given their dehydrating qualities.

- Eat a balanced diet that provides the full spectrum of vitamins and minerals, especially vitamin B and iron.

- Use organic lipsticks that get their pigment from natural sources, such as iron oxides.

- Use a soft children's toothbrush to brush your lips. This removes dead skin and increases blood circulation to the area.

- Heal chapped lips with organic lip balms made from natural emollients such as vegetable oils, natural waxes, or cocoa butter. You can also use a dab of sweet-almond, olive, or coconut oil. Make sure your lip balm has a sunscreen of at least SPF 15.

Don't Gum Up the Works

It's said that the longer we keep our natural teeth, the longer our life span. Holding onto your original teeth depends largely on gum health. Genetics aside, tooth and gum problems are usually rooted in lack of good care. Regular brushing and flossing is one of the best preventives for gum disease, which allows oral bacteria to enter your bloodstream, potentially narrowing your blood vessels, increasing blood clots, and putting you at risk for a heart attack. So love your heart by brushing and flossing at least twice a day. Visit your dentist once a year; twice is even better!

Always brush your teeth after eating, for the health reasons just mentioned and the benefit of clean teeth and fresh breath when interacting with others. Use small, circular motions, spending about three minutes on your full set of choppers. Be gentle! Aggressive brushing creates problems, especially receding gums. Dentists recommend soft, nylon bristles instead of natural bristles, which are usually hard and injure the gums. Use natural, herbal toothpastes, powders, and mouthwashes. Here are but a few of the healthful ingredients to look for on the labels: bloodroot, echinacea, goldenseal, green tea, and myrrh.

You can also make your own bacteria-fighting toothpaste and mouthwash. Mix a thick paste of baking soda and hydrogen peroxide. Add a drop of peppermint essential oil for taste. Follow brushing by rinsing with 1 teaspoon of sea salt dissolved in 8 ounces of warm water. For a mouthwash, add a drop of peppermint essential oil to 1 ounce of water. Also, floss for at least a minute or two every day. Look for natural flosses with cinnamon or tea tree oil, both good for their antibacterial qualities.

And get this! Strawberries have a natural cleansing and bleaching effect, and, in a pinch, provide a great alternative to brushing, such as when you're camping. Crush a strawberry and gently massage the pulp over your teeth. Rinse afterward.

For fresh breath, try chewing on fennel seeds, parsley, or natural mints, or use a natural breath spray. Look for products containing cinnamon, echinacea, tea tree oil, and peppermint to control bacteria while freshening the breath.

Scraping your tongue in the morning reduces bad breath and plaque by eradicating bacteria buildup. Tongue scrapers are widely available these days. You can also brush your tongue, but be gentle.

However, a tongue scraper won't elicit the gag reflex as a toothbrush can.

Saliva Is Important

A cleansing flow of saliva is important for good oral health, because a dry mouth promotes decay. If your saliva flow is negligible, you're undergoing radiation treatments, or you're using drugs that dry your mouth out, speak to you doctor. One of the best natural solutions is to sip water throughout the day or just swish it around in your mouth to rehydrate.

Chewing gum made with parsley-seed oil, sunflower oil, spearmint oil, or the natural sweetener xylitol can help keep saliva flow healthy. Chewing these natural gums after every meal also helps flush away cavity-causing bacteria, sugars, and acids.

Massage for the Mouth

Massage can be as good for your mouth as for the rest of your body. Every day, place a bit of olive or sesame oil on the pad of your finger and gently massage all gum surfaces. This is simply tremendous for stimulating healthy blood flow to the gums. A healthy, organic, unrefined diet with plenty of raw foods and roughage literally helps massage the gums as you chew. Think how your mouth feels after having that apple at the end of your lunch.

You can also activate blood and lymph circulation in your mouth and face muscles by exercising your face. Here are three good ways to do this:

- Twitch your nose back and forth.
- Puff your cheeks out and breathe deeply through your nose ten times. Release and relax your cheeks.
- Do the lion pose from yoga, which has you stretch your mouth wide open, open your eyes all the way, and stick your tongue out as far as it will go. Release and relax. Doing it while looking in the mirror tunes you in to the silliness of the pose, bringing on the laughter.

BEAUTIFUL HANDS AND FEET

The sense organ of touch is our skin and, by extension, our hands and feet. Our hands and feet put us in physical touch with the world. Giving them love and attention will make your whole body feel good. Reflexology and acupressure give us an intimate understanding of this connection. We affect the vitality of every organ and gland, and the body's energy, when we know how and where to touch specific areas on the palms of our hands and soles of our feet. In fact, massaging these wonderful and loyal body parts is so important that we'll explore specific applications for each.

Conscious Care of Our Hands

You largely experience your sense of touch through your hands, like giving yourself or your loved one a massage, running your hands through a loved one's hair, hugging someone dear, stroking your pet's glossy fur, or feeling the silky touch of your bathrobe.

Life flows from our hands into action. As extensions of our heart center, our hands carry out our heartfelt desires. As messengers of our emotions, they help us express our love. As extensions of our work, they perform a staggering amount of functions. Our hands are incredibly sensitive and distinctive. Your fingerprint belongs to you alone. Your palm displays your heart, head, and life lines, and hence your destiny. Spiritualists see the hand as a direct energetic connection to your soul and psyche.

Hand Yoga

Our hands work hard for us and, after a long day, can become achy, as if each of the hand's twenty-seven small bones, thirty joints, and thirty-seven muscles is crying for help. Addressing these little pains now helps you avoid bigger problems later, such as arthritis, tendonitis, carpal tunnel syndrome, and any of the other repetitive-stress injuries. If any part of your body deserves the white-glove treatment, it's your hands.

Like warming up the muscles before launching into full-body exercise, consider warming up and stretching your hands before beginning your day. Try to stretch your hands throughout the day, and stay mindful of how you sit and stand. Poor posture sometimes causes hand discomfort, straining your back, neck, and shoulders, which ultimately can affect your arms, hands, and fingers. For instance, carpal tunnel syndrome is swelling of the tunnel just below the wrist, which pinches the median nerve as it passes through the wrist. It's often caused by repetitive wrist movement, a particularly unnatural or awkward posture, or misaligned vertebrae in the neck.

The best way to prevent repetitive-stress injury is vigilance in changing your body and hand position during repetitive tasks. Also take stretch breaks every ten to fifteen minutes. Doing a few healthy hand stretches throughout the day is also a good idea. Here are a few to consider:

- Interlock your fingers with your palms facing away from you, and stretch your arms as far out in front of you as they'll go. Feel the lovely stretch throughout your hands and arms.

- Chinese harmony balls, also called "health spheres," reduce stress and stimulate your hand's acupressure points, muscles, and nerves. They improve blood circulation and energy flow through your hands and arms, building strength and flexibility. Place the two balls in one hand and revolve them around each other as long as you want. Also listen to their melodic sound.

- Stress-relief or grip-strengthener balls provide many of the same benefits as Chinese harmony balls. Keep them in your desk drawer, next to the bed or TV, and in your car. These simple devices work great for stress relief and developing hand and forearm strength.

Also try this hand yoga sequence for maintaining full range of motion:

1. Place your right elbow on a flat surface, with your right palm facing you.

2. Place your left wrist on your right palm. Let gravity take over as your left arm hangs there.

3. Breathe deeply several times, and then gently arch your right wrist up, in the opposite direction to that it was hanging in. This counters the first powerful stretch.

4. Repeat this sequence on the other side, with your left hand supporting your right wrist.

5. Again place your right elbow on a flat surface with your palm facing toward you.

6. Using the index and middle fingers on your left hand, hang onto the thumb of your right hand. Feel the stretch through your palm and wrist.

7. Take several deep breaths. Bend your right fingers inward to counter the previous stretch.

8. Repeat this sequence on the other side to stretch your left palm and wrist.

Performed at intervals through the day, these two stretches benefit strained hand tendons and muscles.

Be Gentle on Your Hands

We all want silky, youthful hands, and we can have them by providing our time and loving attention. Nutrition and physical activity are important to optimize blood circulation and deliver nutrients to our skin. Externally, we want to practice diligence in protecting our hands. Keep natural hand-washing liquid and nourishing moisturizer at every sink in the house. Carry a small container of moisturizer with you. While working the moisturizer in, give yourself a mini hand massage. Be present and send healing energy to yourself. Breathe deeply. Stroke, gently roll, and "milk" the fingers from base to tip, easing the joints. Massage with small, circular strokes through your palm. Apply pressure to the web area between each finger, lingering between the thumb and index finger, a powerful acupressure point (the *hoku* point) for alleviating fatigue and pain. Now move to the soft tissue between the tendons and bones on the back of your hand, working toward the wrist, increasing blood and energy flow.

Make it a habit to moisturize your hands often during the day, and especially at bedtime! This is the most effective way to preserve and shield your hands from environmental stressors.

Here are a few more strategies to keep your hands happy and healthy:

- Have a professional hand treatment in tandem with a manicure. Professional nail technicians and massage therapists offer hand and foot massages that are as relaxing as they are beautifying.

- A soak in sea salt or Epsom salts can be quite helpful if your hands are swollen or sore.

- For hands as smooth as silk, soak them in warm milk for five to ten minutes.

- Use calendula or chamomile essential oil to nourish and moisturize the skin of the hands by adding two to three drops to either a warm-water hand soak or the hand lotion or plant oil you use to moisturize and massage your hands.

- Smear organic honey, one of nature's best moisturizers, over your hands and relax for ten to fifteen minutes. When you're ready, rinse your hands with warm water (gentle soap is optional).

- Be sure to use body-exfoliating product on your hands too to encourage sloughing off of dead skin cells and cellular turnover.

- Wear gloves whenever appropriate to prevent harming your hands, such as when gardening, in very cold weather, or when washing dishes.

Conscious Care for Your Feet

Leonardo da Vinci described feet as a masterpiece of engineering and a work of art. Our feet keep us grounded to the earth's energies while taking us where we want to go. Ah, what faithful servants our feet are! It's only fitting that we treat them with the care and attention they so richly deserve.

The foot contains twenty-six bones, thirty-three joints, nineteen muscles, and one hundred-seven ligaments. Virtually supporting the entire body, feet tend to reflect the state of your mind and heart. If you don't believe me, consider the endless foot metaphors to describe our moods and inclinations. When decisive, self-confident, flexible, and on the move, we're fleet of foot or quick on our feet. When immobilized, weak, or wishy-washy, we have feet of clay or are dragging our feet. We get a foot up on our business competitors, and our dogs howl after a day of rushing around. So to put your best foot forward, start taking care of those feet today.

Here are some great ways to nurture your feet:

- Take a footbath using essential oils with toning, astringent, and antiseptic properties, such as eucalyptus, juniper, lavender, rosemary, and tea tree. Add two to six drops to a container filled with warm water. Along with the soothing and stimulating qualities of these oils, their toning properties firm foot skin tissue, reducing the amount of oil and perspiration excreted from the skin. The antiseptic quality helps with odor issues. This footbath balances the amount of foot perspiration expelled, washes away sweat, and refreshes your feet—and your mind! Anyone can use it anytime.

- Soak your feet in a bath infused with black tea. Brew two tea bags in two pints of water, and then add two quarts of cool water. The tannic acid acts as a drying agent and helps prevent odor.

- Many spas provide a delightful footbath and scrub ritual as a prelude to any service. When your feet need a little TLC, give them a warm-water soak. A soak can soothe, smooth, protect, and stabilize your feet. (It's also a great preparatory step before massaging your feet.) Add Epsom or sea salts (natural exfoliants), which help relax the feet and soften any rough, dry patches of skin. You can also add one to two cups of pure pineapple juice; an enzyme in the juice (bromelain) naturally sloughs off dry skin. Or, try mixing a tablespoon of sea salt with a tablespoon of sweet-almond oil. Soak (or shower or bathe) to soften skin, then scrub callused areas for a few minutes with this mixture. Scrubbing with a pumice stone and a gentle body wash removes dry, rough, or calloused skin. Rinse, towel off, moisturize, and then don fluffy organic-cotton socks.

It's a long way from your heart to the tips of your toes, but for healthy, comfortable feet, it's important to encourage blood flow to them. Both exercise and massage play important roles. Also, choose well-fitting shoes. Forfeiting comfort for style might look great, but the repercussions will have you walking a painful path, possibly filled with bunions, calluses, plantar fasciitis, deformed toes, and various other potential maladies.

Exercise Those Tootsies!

Exercise is essential for maintaining the mobility and flexibility of your feet. Foot exercises may also relieve soreness, particularly if you have flat feet. Naturally, see a podiatrist when warranted, but here are a few exercises you can do anytime, anywhere:

- Rock back and forth from your heels to your toes for several minutes.

- Try picking up marbles with your toes.

- Lay a towel flat on the floor. Scrunch your toes up on the towel, drawing the fabric toward you.

- Roll your arches over a tennis ball, golf ball, or rolling pin.

- Revisit tadasana (mountain pose) for its foot-rejuvenating benefits. Lift your toes and spread them open wide before planting them into the earth. Also, yoga sandals are now available that have spacers that separate each toe. They're awesome!

Foot Massage

Massage is such a treat for your feet; it encourages better blood flow to this area, and just plain feels good. We've already addressed how massaging your feet every night before turning in produces profound relaxation. When you release tension in your feet, your mind-body physiology is sure to follow. Use a small amount of certified-organic plant oil or lotion with several drops of geranium, lavender, patchouli, or tea tree essential oil, all of which possess potent antibacterial effects. These ingredients are also in many store-bought preparations.

Begin your foot massage by distributing massage oil or lotion through the hands. Briskly stroke the soles, and go on to massage the rest of your feet with a combination of small strokes. Use smaller strokes between the bones along the top of your foot, working toward your ankle, and thus your heart, which is important for directing blood flow. Gently pull each toe outward from base to tip. Put on organic-cotton socks, and it's time for bed! Doing this every night for the rest of your life is a stabilizing and healthful part of your daily routine that will render your feet absolutely beautiful to behold.

Also, look for the wonderful foot lotions that contain my all-time-favorite ingredient for cooling off and reviving stressed or hot feet—peppermint essential oil.

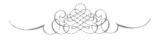

CONCLUSION

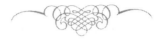

KNOWING OURSELVES AS BEAUTIFUL

Let the beauty we love be what we do.

—RUMI, THIRTEENTH-CENTURY PERSIAN POET

We've been hanging out together throughout this book: I've shared my soul, and I hope you've gotten fully involved—and loved every moment of the pleasure *and* the healing! You hold the magic, the transformative power to create exquisite wholeness in your life, and when you do, you ignite that spark we mentioned earlier, casting a beautiful glow on everyone and everything you encounter. Can you see this in your mind's eye? Do you see how your internal synergy becomes the world's synergy?

As the Oracle at Delphi said, "Know thyself." Always know that you can trust your inner sense to guide you to make the most life-affirming and holistic choices possible. As you find a deeper understanding of your authentic self and your purpose in life, you become the very best you can be.

So choose your dreams, goals, and values; then go forward to plan and enact. Spirit will guide you, but you need to stay in touch with spirit for this to happen. The eternal self is just waiting to be joyfully nurtured into existence. Ah, self-creation—your true purpose in life. "Creating" yourself, or nurturing yourself into an existence you proudly love, can involve the smallest act of loving-kindness or the largest undertaking of detoxifying the world. It can entail an earthly experience or something of an entirely spiritual nature. As you tap into the pure-consciousness layer of your being, you'll radiate synergy—and your light will shine. You'll realize that you're more beautiful, brilliant, creative, and loving than you even imagined. You're here to manifest this divinity within you.

Become truly centered in your being. May we all practice being still and really listening to ourselves, each other, and the gentle intelligence of the living earth. Doing so builds the contagious energy that leads to renewal, rejuvenation, and rebirth, to real healing and restoration of our wholeness as individuals and a global community, fostering our deep interdependence among humankind and with every species, as well as the whole interwoven web of creation.

This is all part of nurturing self, because in this we continue to grow, as we follow our path toward self-realization. This is all part of the same thing, your evolutionary consciousness. Every one of us is on an evolutionary arc that will bring us all home to the same state of being in the end. Be as gentle, kind, and loving as you can. Know that finding challenges along this path is a sign that you're taking responsibility for yourself, others, and the earth. Growing more aware of what you do makes you an active participant in, and witness to, one of the most important paradigm shifts taking place in modern times. "Think globally, act locally" never rang more true than today. Don't feel as if any of your actions are ever inconsequential, especially in view of the immense challenges we face in our times. Any action you take toward healing yourself or your world is significant in the overall cumulative result of millions of others also making small changes in their lives; it's a collective consciousness. The character of our entire society is changing dramatically because of the collective and transformative ripple effect of each wave in the ocean of humanity. Our flow through the wholeness of life is founded on unity within ourselves, with others, and with Mother Earth. Together, let's embed ourselves in the sacredness, unity, and sensuousness of nature, our own and that surrounding us. Truly, there can be no finer seduction than surrounding yourself with beauty and living a holistic, sustainable, healing lifestyle—all with great pleasure! This is the true spirit of well-being. Yes, you've now embarked on a spiritual quest that permeates every facet of your life and being. Plunge in, immerse yourself, and be seduced by the ecstasy of it all!

References

Arnot, B. 2000. Alter your biology to create sizzling mental energy. *USA Weekend*, January 16. http://www.usaweekend.com/00_issues/000116/000116biology.html.

Association for Applied and Therapeutic Humor. What everyone should know about humor and laughter. http://www.aath.org/documents/AATH-WhatWeKnowREVISED.pdf, accessed January 15, 2005.

Berk, L. 1996. Interview in Humor and Health Journal, September/October. Summary at Holisticonline.com, Humor section, http://holisticonline.com/Humor_Therapy/humor_therapy_benefits.htm.

Gilda's Club Chicago. 2003. Laughter convention comes to Chicago co-sponsored by Gilda's Club Chicago. February 11 http://www.gildasclubchicago.org/news/.

Miller, H. 1939. *Tropic of Capricorn*. New York: Grove Press, Inc., 1994.

Neimark, J. 1997. Mind body: Mystical connection—How Candace Pert, neuroscientist and alternative medicine guru, discovered the body's natural opiates, known as endorphins. *Psychology Today*, November–December. http://psychologytoday.com/articles/pto-19971101-000026.html.

Pert, C. B. 1997. *Molecules of Emotion: Why You Feel the Way You Feel.* New York: Scribner.

Seaward, B. L. 1997. *Managing Stress: Principles and Strategies for Health and Well-Being.* 2nd ed. Boston: Jones and Bartlett Publishers.

"*Pleasure Healing* is a joy to read. I can think of no better compliment than to say I'd like to have written it myself! Mary Beth Janssen has given those in search of a healthier, more fulfilling life a roadmap that is both inspiring and practical. Turning these pages is a spa journey in itself—a beautiful release from distraction and worry guided by an author who is intuitive and wise."

—Deborah Szekely, cofounder of Rancho La Puerta with her husband Edmond Szekely, and founder of the Golden Door Spa

"*Pleasure Healing* promises to create transformational change in your life through conscious living and loving of self and others. You create this change through your attention and intention, becoming the decision-maker to bring vitality, joy, compassion and creativity into your life. Mary Beth takes you on a mindful journey through several healing rituals, and I highly recommend her holistic approach."

—Gay Hendricks, Ph.D., author of *Five Wishes* and coauthor, with Kathlyn Hendricks, Ph.D., of *Conscious Loving*

"*Pleasure Healing* offers sound advice for anyone who is willing to have less stress and more joy, laughter, and balance in their life."

—Arielle Ford, author of *The Soulmate Secret* and the *Hot Chocolate for the Mystical Soul* book series

"In this book, Janssen uses her big heart and wealth of knowledge to inspire people to live their greatest lives. Pleasure Healing is an amazing resource for those seeking two powerful experiences: pleasure and healing."

—Max Simon, founder and CEO of Selfcentered Meditation